I dedicate this book to my truly inspirational and supportive wife and my fantastic daughter

Table of Contents

Chapter 1: Cancer Briefly Explained 6

Chapter 2: Introductory Diet Advice 15

Chapter 3: Mediterranean Diet & Super Herbs 24

Chapter 4: Vitamin A, C, D, E & Selenium 48

Chapter 5: Almonds 61

Chapter 6: The Tomato or Golden Apple 66

Chapter 7: What is Oxidative Stress?. 77

Chapter 8: Oxidative Stress & Enzymes 100

Chapter 9: Aspirin & Other Anti-inflammatories 128

Chapter 10: Placebo Effect 147

Chapter 11: Laughter 154

Chapter 12: Pineapple's - Bromelian 166

Chapter 13: Broccoli & Cruciferous Vegetables 170

Chapter 14: Homeopathic Condurango, Arsenicum Album & Ruta Graveolens 176

Chapter 15: Turmeric, Black Pepper & Red Chilli Peppers 183

References 192

IMPORTANT INTRODUCTION – Fight Cancer in 60 days – A scientific and holistic approach

First I would like to talk briefly about cancer and the approach that this book takes regarding it. It is not my objective for people to reject modern medical, radiological and surgical procedures in their fight against cancer but to attempt to compliment it. Traditional cancer care has its successes and failures and lack of scientific agreement internationally. I will discuss a wide range of ideas that have been scientifically researched although not necessarily agreed upon and give you my thoughts on them. I feel that there is a good scientific evidence base which is often ignored or not given enough weight, credence or promotion for many reasons, often financial, other than scientific rigor or validity. I am a registered clinical physiologist and healthcare scientist not a doctor and so do not intend for you to take any advice given without first consulting your own doctor as to its likely impact on your current condition and treatment. I have personally experienced stage IV cancer over 30 years ago and also seen its effects on friends, family and patients. During my own journey I was intrigued how traditional surgical, radiological and chemotherapeutic medicine often dismissed complementary medicine as invalidated. However I was lucky to be treated extremely well by a truly capable and enlightened oncologist Dr. C. J. Tyrrell who was not dismissive at that time but said it was worth reviewing the science but keeping him informed of any changes I intended to make to my diet etc. My mother and wife have been inspirational in the benefits of a healthy diet and my interest in this area. Even though I am well now I continued to research this area to help others. I expect you to consider your own body and review a range of sources before making your own grown-up decision and acting on it and accepting your responsibility for your actions. Obviously if you are unable to do that please give this book away and do something more constructive or fun with your time.

Cancer is a major health concern and impacts on the majority of us either directly or indirectly. Cancer is the second leading cause of death due to ill health in the USA with first place going to cardiovascular ("heart") disease. It seems both conditions have similarities and are loosely linked by their pathophysiology apart from their ability to kill. These similarities are why certain treatments can affect both disease processes in a physiological manner, particularly those involving inflammation and epithelial cells. Clearly cancer in someone with other severe health conditions can lead to a poorer outcome or prognosis and equally a healthy heart is certainly going to help the body overcome certain severe health conditions such as cancer.

It is important if you are pregnant or ill to be exceptionally careful with anything you eat or drink or do and so please like everyone else do nothing discussed in this book without consulting your doctor.

It is hoped by following the homework jobs-to-do plan discussed in this book in consultation with your oncologist that ideally in combination with your health plan from your oncologist you should sustain a noticeable benefit to your health. Clearly this cannot be guaranteed and proved individually, as the cause of any growth or reduction in tumours is subject to many variables as with all forms of healthcare. The information and suggestions are put forward with some supporting scientific ideas however healthcare for cancer and especially nutritional care are not an exact proven science with guaranteed results.

The scientific references used to formulate ideas are at the end of this book, if you wish to do further in depth reading about each area. Many of the scientific papers can be accessed in full online and will go into far more detail that the overview presented in this book.

Important advice to reader: *Do read this introduction again but do not feel compelled to read the rest of this book in any particular order as it is organized so that you can read a chapter independently. You will still gain some useful information which may help you, a family member or a friend in the fight against cancer. Oxidative stress is a major factor in chronic inflammation and many cancers and is good to understand. Chapters 7, 8 & 9 are particularly heavy going especially in one go, as they attempt to explain oxidative stress in some scientific detail, so if getting a headache may be read 7 and then skip to Chapter 10 and then back to 8 again and then skip to Chapter 11 and so forth.*

*All suggestions under the **Jobs to Do** headings are obviously just suggestions and not medical advice but personal decisions you make after discussion with your oncologist.*

Chapter 1: Cancer Briefly Explained

What follows is a brief and straight-forward discussion about cancer. It is deliberately limited as this book is primarily to help you in your fight against cancer and not to give you "War and Peace" type details on the condition. Having said that it does help to know your enemy in any fight and so with that in mind what follows is a brief overview. There is a wealth of more detailed information explaining cancer elsewhere if required.

Many types of cancer can be prevented to a degree, such as those caused by environmental factors e.g. smoking. Now many cancers if diagnosed early can be treated with good results using modern medicine provided in a hospital environment.

There are very many theories about why cells become cancerous and their division and growth become accelerated. Some are now obvious such as external toxins or irritants (e.g. cigarette smoke or coal dust), but others are less clear such as bacterially or virally stimulated, inherited or internal DNA damage.

There are clearly physiological relations between all theories such as the damage done to cells by excessive oxidative stress, which is explained in some detail in this book. It is important to realise that not only do cancerous cells grow and divide rapidly, but that they do not die naturally and so like a snowball running down a hill in a cartoon they can get bigger and bigger and bigger without treatment. It is just a matter of time and type how big they become. For example a so-called benign cancer (not so "dangerous") is often slower growing and doesn't spread but can still cause damage. They can cause damage to normal cell function in their vicinity but also interfere with body functions. A good example is cancer of the kidney, which can interfere with the normal working of the kidney. Some cancerous cells can also spread (metastasize.) to other parts of the body and cause a cancerous growth and damage in another area. There are other cancers such as leukaemia where no specific tumour is caused but the cancerous cells cause damage to the normal functioning of blood and bone marrow. Cancers are generally named after the place where they first started, for example a cancer in the lung which started in the prostrate gland would still be called prostrate cancer. Cancer usually occurs due to genetic damage that happens inside a single cell. This cell is often called a malignant cell. These malignant cells generally divide much more quickly than normal cells. It is during this active dividing stage that most anticancer drugs act. This is why with some chemotherapy drugs patients' hair falls out, because hair follicle cells normally divide rapidly as well as malignant cells.

We tend to say the word cancer as if it were a single condition but in fact there are more than a hundred different and separate types of cancers. It therefore follows that one type of treatment is unlikely to cure all these different types. These different types do have similar characteristics in that they all have abnormal and uncontrolled cell growth. The growing ball of cells or tumour is maintained by nutrients from the blood system and can even cause for its own use, little specialized mini blood system to form so that blood vessels are formed (angiogenesis) to feed the growth of the tumour. This occurrence can be very helpful to aid diagnosis and therefore treatment. In general the damage that cancer causes can be by direct or indirect means. That is indirectly its growth in a restricted area can exert pressure on nearby cells and organs thus affecting their physiology or ability to function or directly by invading tissue or organs or by its toxins affecting their physiology or ability to function. In healthy people cells tend to grow, divide, and eventually die in a standard and predictable way. This natural cell death process is often called normal programmed cell death or apoptosis. There are changes in how cells act throughout our normal lives, for example as a child normal cells will grow and divide quicker as we grow. Once we are adult size our cell numbers don't increase much as cells generally only divide and grow to replace old or damaged ones. This is a sort of maintenance phase to cover general wear and tear.

The growing ball of cells known as cancer can destroy surrounding cells and body tissues and may even spread to other parts of the body. This occurs when malignant cells are released into the blood system usually. Although cancer cells are part of your own body they often act like a parasite or foreign body only interested in their own survival. Luckily your body sometimes recognizes cancerous cells as unusual and tries to do battle with these cells. Many malignant cells die due to the physical nature of being battered about within the circulatory system and level of blood pressure, whilst others are killed by the superheroes of our blood system the White Blood Cells and our immune system in general.

There are really three main means that cancer is treated using traditional styles of medicine although many medical doctors are now also looking at incorporating complimentary therapies as part of their treatment plans in a more standardized way. The three main treatment pathways include surgery ("cutting the cancer out"), radiotherapy ("blasting the cancer with radiation") and chemotherapy ("killing the cancer with powerful drugs"). There have been tremendous advances in all of these over the past decades especially in recent years. Effectiveness and reduction in side effects have improved but still the prognosis and side effects for some treatments and some cancers could be improved. Side effects such as nausea, gastric discomfort, hair loss, fatigue, poor blood clotting, reduced immune system, anemia, loss of appetite and pain still occur. These are explained to you for your specific cancer or treatment generally if predictable and how to best manage them. I will focus on things that I believe will help reduce the effect of these side effects as well as help in your fight against cancer.

We can see that the immune system and general body physiology is highly important especially when linked with a healthy cardiovascular and blood system. Throughout this book we will look at areas that impact on the physiology of the body and enable it to better fight cancer.

Radiotherapy
I am not going to go into great detail for this area because the focus of the book is how you can improve your own chances of surviving cancer and not how traditional medical treatments can. However I think in addition to re-stating that major advances in healthcare have occurred in recent years with the associated increase in survival rates, it is also useful to briefly discuss new and different treatment regimes available. A very important way of helping your survival is to not assume that you are receiving the latest available or best treatment. Perceptions of the best form of therapy will vary from cancer to cancer and from doctor to doctor and from country to country. A certain degree of trust is implicit with all healthcare but a high level is especially necessary for cancer care. **This does not stop you from obtaining a second opinion from another doctor. This will help you accept or not a particular diagnosis but also help you trust that the treatment offered is the best medical treatment available or not.**

It is now well over a century since the German physicist, Wilhelm Conrad Roentgen, discovered X-rays and took the first human x-ray "picture", which was one of his wife's left hand. Months later one of the first to use X-ray radiation to treat cancer was in fact a Chicago chemist and homeopathic physician named Émil Grubbé (1875-1960) in 1896. After x-raying his own hand several times and suffering severe damage he realised that something so powerful if used in minute doses according to homeopathic law might actually heal severe illness. He trialled it on one of the first recorded patients a 55-

year old woman suffering from recurrent and then inoperable breast cancer after radical mastectomy, although she died soon after the race was on to perfect the process. Following on from this, the ground-breaking research of Marie Curie and others showed that radiation could be used not only to help diagnosis, but to help treat cancer (radiotherapy) and if excess exposure occurs in fact cause cancer.

In the UK and many other countries traditional medical cancer care consists of surgery, chemotherapy or radiotherapy and often a combination of these treatments. Generally chemotherapy, that is treating cancer with drugs, is considered by many preferable due to the increased general radiation dose received with radiotherapy. However both methods have unwanted side-effects and so often the decision of which form of therapy to use is more related to relative success of the therapy for a particular cancer. The research discussed and "advice" throughout this book should not only help you fight cancer whilst complimenting traditional medical cancer care but should help you also fight some of the significant side-effects of radiotherapy and chemotherapy.

In terms of success rate comparisons, surgery and radiotherapy are often the most effective treatments for cancers especially in adults. Radiotherapy has progressed significantly in recent years with millions of people being successfully treated each year with very few side-effects. Research still continues in most countries with **Cancer** Research UK, and the Medical Research Council working together in the UK to improve radiotherapy success. Unfortunately although in many ways the UK leads the world in research due to the way healthcare is funded in the UK, these research advances are not translated widely into clinical benefits for the majority, i.e. you may not get the very latest laser radiotherapy treatment in the majority of the UK. It is important to remember also that the latest does not always equal the best treatment.

However recent exciting advances in radiotherapy that are being clinically used widely in the USA and other wealthy countries are not clinically used so widely in the UK at the time of writing. I am referring to proton therapy which delivers much more targeted radiotherapy. This means that the tumour is treated far more effectively and there is less likelihood of damage to the healthy surrounding tissue. A recent systematic review by a Dutch team of researchers looked at the effectiveness of carbon-ion, proton and photon radiotherapy for head and neck cancer. The team reviewed a number of aspects including symptom improvements, survival and toxic side-effects. It appeared that photon therapy was the most commonly used treatment although not proved to be the most effective. This seemed to be for a mixture of reasons such as its evidence-base but also physicians' training and the status quo. Proton therapy is helping to reduce unnecessary long-term damage and side-effects. I strongly recommend you talk with your doctor about whether there are other forms of treatment available in the USA or other wealthy countries which are successful for your form of cancer but not available in the UK through the NHS.

Due to improved imaging techniques it is now possible to pinpoint cancers more accurately, that is to within millimetres. There are also advances in using ultrasound to treat cancers. A therapy named focal therapy uses High Intensity Focused Ultrasound which focuses ultrasound on the tumour itself in a similar way to proton therapy such that the tumour is treated far more effectively and there is less likelihood of damage to the healthy surrounding tissue and associated side-effects. The technique is discussed in a scientific paper on the clinical implications of this therapy in the *New England Journal of Medicine*. Dr Ahmed states that for prostrate cancer it focuses on "ablation of only the malignant areas within the prostate, along with a margin of normal tissue, and preservation of normal prostate and surrounding structures will help reduce side effects."

It is relatively early days for clinical use of this therapy and only limited long-term data is available, but it seems that this technique maybe successful. In fact it may be just as successful as the standard surgical removal of the whole gland but without many of the unwanted side-effects. These side-effects are not insignificant in terms of quality of life long after treatment and can include impotence and incontinence. It is also hoped that this treatment will be more specific and focused and thus help stop the spread of additional cancers (metastases) from the original cancer core.

Regular Intensity Modulated RadioTherapy (IMRT) uses photons and for many cancers can help with significant survival of cancer. Although for effective tumour control the radiation doses are high. This also means higher radiation doses for healthy tissues with the associated increased risks of toxicity. Some recent studies have shown that radiotherapy using high-energy proton beams can deliver highly focused doses to the cancerous tissue whilst reducing the dose delivered to nearby healthy tissues compared to standard IMRT. During standard IMRT not only is local healthy tissue exposed to radiation from the main beam which has been scattered within the patient to some degree, but also healthy tissue not in the local area are exposed to general leakage radiation from the machine. This undesired radiation of healthy tissue means that patients receiving this have over their life a small increase in risk of developing a second cancer as a result of the radiation. It is therefore anticipated that patients receiving proton therapy will have lower overall radiation exposure and therefore less risk of a second cancer caused by excessive radiation. There is not full agreement with this idea yet by the clinical or research communities as there is little hard evidence which agrees with the International Commission on Radiological Protection protocols.

It is worth being aware that proton therapy although gaining more widespread use is far from new. In fact proton therapy was first used for treating cancer over 40 years ago in the USA at Massachusetts General Hospital. Proton therapy has over the years been enhanced and more focussed. The proton dose is delivered in a very focussed way with no general radiation dose being delivered more than a few millimetres away. There have been studies reviewing the various benefits of proton therapy over regular IMRT for certain cancers and there are obviously still limited detailed longitudinal studies. It would appear for cancers which are confined to specific centres and where sparing healthy tissue is considered important there has been some worthwhile success. Cancers of the face, brain, spine and prostrate have seen worthwhile healthy tissue survival and successful treatment of the cancer. I am sure that as time passes that proton therapy will become a more significant tool in the treatment of cancer.

We have focused on primarily radiotherapy this chapter but it is important to state that chemotherapy is very successful and equally progressive. Clearly there are always going to be advances in the field of modern science and when dealing with your health and ultimately your long term life, it is important that care and due thought take place before decisions are made. Your cancer and how you fight it are individual to you and clearly you should try to seek appropriate medical information and guidance as previously stated and maybe even from several doctors to ensure you obtain the best form of treatment from traditional sources.

Jobs to do

I think you have probably guessed this one already but it really can be a major step in fighting your cancer. There are many cases where people have done just this one job and had significantly improved treatment, increased remission and survival projections let alone improved quality of life after treatment.

> 1. Make an appointment and ask your doctor if there are other treatments available which are not supported by the NHS which are widely respected elsewhere such as USA, Germany or research programmes. If not happy generally with the information or care package planned for you then as with all healthcare seek a second opinion or more. It is important to add that you do not want to unnecessarily extend the decision-making process to the extent that you start no treatment of any kind as most often in cancer timely supported treatment leads to better outcomes.

Chapter 2: Introductory Diet Advice & Surprise Finding - A healthy diet & exercise are important

Traditional cancer treatments such as surgery and radiotherapy but especially chemotherapy are very powerful tools in the fight against cancer but are widely considered very blunt tools. Many people believe this is because of the collateral damage these treatments do to the body's organs and physiological processes not suffering from cancer. It has been seen in the past that this aggressive approach means that a patient can be cured of cancer but still die due to the damage done to the body by the process of attempted cure. For example past cancer survivors receiving large doses of chemotherapy have died after the "cure" because of pneumonia due to a severely damaged and less effective immune system.

Symptoms such as problems with the digestive tract (digestion and absorption), fatigue, severe loss of appetite, feeling full and changes in taste and smell are common side effects of cancer treatment, which can lead to poor nutrition and even malnutrition. Significant drops in weight and poor nutrition are noted in more than half the patients diagnosed with cancer. It is therefore essential that keeping active and well fed is part of any cancer fighter's health regime as any further weight loss is likely to lead to a poor recovery. Clearly if possible exercise and additional protein shakes with supplements can be beneficial if weight loss is present or likely to occur. Ideally get referred to your own specialist dietician / nutritionist who will individually tailor a diet to your actual needs rather than general advice.

By drinking less alcohol and having many little meals taken more often is a way many patients find it possible to maintain their required food intake to reduce weight loss. There are many studies that show majorly improved outcomes for people who receive dietary consultations during treatment. The improved outcomes include less weight loss and fewer negative side-effects from the traditional treatments. The fear of having to receive food and fluid via a tube is usually enough to focus most people's mind regarding eating the right amount with help but sometimes for the very mal-nourished and ill this method of feeding is essential for survival.

The use of dietary and vitamin supplements is often very useful. You should always discuss their use with your doctor as some can interact with cancer drugs. Many cancer fighters take dietary supplements that contain high levels of antioxidants (e.g. vitamins C and E). The levels taken often far exceed the daily recommended amount for healthy adults, but because cancer fighters are far from healthy adults, they feel the benefits far outweigh any risks. It is likely that there are often real benefits in helping protect normal cells from the collateral damage caused by traditional treatments.

Many researchers have looked at the benefits of exercise during cancer treatment. Most studies are a bit limited but the majority, not unsurprisingly recommend that exercise is safe and beneficial during cancer treatment. The benefits relate to improved physiological function, overall health and appetite as well as an improved sense of well-being. Exercise has been shown to improve heart function, muscle strength, body mass, fatigue, anxiety, depression, self-esteem, happiness, and several components of quality of life (physical, functional, and emotional) and importantly longevity in cancer fighters.

A degree of commonsense is required in that for most people this does not mean extreme exercise will aid the fight against cancer more or is desirable during or following treatment but moderate-to-vigorous physical activity can help in the fight against cancer due to its physiological benefits such as aiding cardiopulmonary fitness and general detoxification. There have been few specific studies, but research among men with prostate cancer who received radiation therapy suggests that men who exercised routinely had significant benefits and fewer side effects to the treatment. I hope it is obvious that running a marathon for the first time after treatment is not going to be a good idea but a gradual approach to exercise and stamina is required. This is especially true for cancer fighters who have not exercised properly for some time and those confined to bed for long periods. If you have suffered from anaemia or very high blood pressure during treatment it is advisable to check that this has been rectified before exercising. Being more active generally is good start for everyone.

Most side-effects to traditional cancer therapies such as nausea are short lived but some are longer lasting. These longer lasting side effects can include life threatening and life altering ones such as anorexia, severe weight loss, changed sense of taste and severely dysfunctional gut leading to regular diarrhoea or constipation. In the long term fight against cancer and its traditional treatment these side effects need to be acted on ideally with the help of a dietician to relieve symptoms and stimulate appetite to aid full recovery. It can be seen that life after traditional cancer treatment needs to be managed properly to help improve not just length of life but also quality of life. This is why many people review their lifestyles and diets to help ensure no re-occurrence of cancer but also to aid full recovery. It also helps with the avoidance of other potentially harmful diseases such as heart disease diabetes, and osteoporosis.

Being fat and lazy is not a healthy choice for cancer fighters. Unfortunately there is plenty of data about significant health risks including cancer from being obese. Equally being too skinny and lazy is also dangerous for cancer fighters.

I do not intend to turn this into a diet book but obviously a healthy diet that balances fat, protein, and carbohydrates appropriately is essential for cancer fighters before, during and after traditional treatment. As a general rule a diet that is similar to those at risk of or suffering from heart disease is indicated. A good rule of thumb for a healthy diet is that 15% is protein, 25% is fat and 60% is carbohydrate.

Fats
There are many studies on diet and cancer but clearly each person's cancer and nutritional needs is individual. Results from studies in the USA and Canada showed that the risk in re-occurrence of breast cancer was reduced by a quarter in women on a low fat diet, whilst the risk of earlier death was three times less for those women on a low fat diet with a greater monounsaturated fat intake. Omega-3 fatty acids seem to have real benefits for cancer fighters following treatment. These benefits include reducing weight loss and muscular wasting and improving treatment outcomes. It is important for cancer fighters to try to include natural sources of these fatty acids wherever possible rather than just taking supplements. Foods that are rich in omega-3 fatty acids include fish and walnuts.

Protein
Good levels of protein intake are essential before, during and after cancer treatment and have been seen to aid long-term survival. The best protein is in foods that are also low in saturated fat such as fish, nuts, seeds, poultry, eggs, low-fat dairy products and even lean red meat if you must. Soy-derived foods are a great source of protein and so a good alternative to most meat. Soy contains many phytochemicals. Some of these phytochemicals act in a similar way to oestrogen, the "female" hormone and can help cancer fighters. It seems especially useful for men with prostate cancer but it may be best to limit intake for women with breast cancer as it could stimulate re-occurrence in high levels.

Carbohydrates
The best carbohydrates are in foods that are rich in essential nutrients, phytochemicals, and fibre, such

as vegetables, fruit, and whole grains. It is best if these foods provide the majority of your carbohydrates. Vegetables and fruits are considered by many the cancer fighters' best friends because not only do they contain fibre which aids digestion but they also contain many active chemicals that often slow cancer progression hence why there are very many fresh juice diets for cancer fighters. Avoid concentrates and go for whole fruit juices. The plant chemicals in fruits and vegetables include essential vitamins and minerals and active phytochemicals. We will discuss some plants and specific chemicals in detail throughout the book. Be careful if you are vegetarian to get plenty of vitamin D ideally from sunlight (not midday sun and in moderation, whilst checking with your doctor for increased risk of skin cancer) not supplements. It is also important if vegetarian to get plenty of calories as vegetables can fill you up but when ill may not sustain your calorific needs.

Plants
In general terms due to our body's and the world's evolution it would appear vegetables of allsorts are recommended to aid our digestion and metabolism. Increasing your overall intake of vegetables and fruits is a great way to reduce the risk of several different cancers such as mouth, throat, stomach and colon cancers.

Some vegetables seem to be more significant in their anti-cancer effects than others. Ones that have been heavily researched and show strong anti-cancer properties are the cruciferous vegetables (such as broccoli and cauliflower) and tomatoes. In general the more colourful vegetables are the better including dark green, red and orange vegetables, which are full of phytochemicals. On the whole fresh is best where possible. Cooking vegetables and fruits by steaming stops the leeching out of important chemicals and aids digestion so is advised over boiling.

Whole grains

Whole grains are rich in chemicals that have important anti-cancer properties. Whole grains include chemicals that have hormonal and antioxidant properties. Whole grains contain antioxidants, such as Vitamin E, phenolic acids, flavonoids, lignans, phytosterols and unsaturated fatty acids. All of these chemicals have been seen to reduce risk and progression of cancer as well as cardiovascular disease.

Sugar

In Great Britain sugar has become the new public health enemy No.1. Excessive refined sugar is not good for you generally but clinically sugar has not been shown to directly increase cancer risk or progression. However the famous biochemist and Nobel Laureate Otto Warburg was convinced that sugar had a direct impact on cancer progression due to cancer cells gaining their energy by non-oxidative breakdown of glucose. He was one of the great scientists of the 20th Century and held in high esteem by Einstein. He in fact gained his Nobel Prize for his ground-breaking work in this area and felt that it was this "fermentation" of glucose by these cells that was the primary cause of cancer. Although more current scientists have argued the case of other causes these he believed and so do others were in fact secondary causes. It seems that now healthcare is slowly changing its view on refined sugar. Personally it seems entirely reasonable to take on board his extensive work and eliminate all forms of refined sugar from your diet whilst fighting cancer. Anecdotally many cancer fighters have felt better for removing it from their diets as they have increased their general diet to fill the gap and have noted improved appetites.

Alcohol

The good news is that alcohol is good for you. The bad news is that it is also bad for you in large amounts. There is plenty of guidance regarding what is considered healthy but I would like to add that you are in charge of your own drinking levels and so if it makes the odd bad day better it is probably a good thing for your morale to break the "rules" once in a while if you like to drink alcohol. Red wine due to its high levels of phytochemicals is considered better than many other alcoholic drinks. Guinness due to its high levels of iron and calories is also good choice for the odd tipple. Alcohol in moderate amounts can lower risk for heart disease, but unfortunately more alcohol does not lower the risk more but has the opposite effect. High levels of alcohol can increase the risk of mouth, throat, liver, breast, and colon cancers

Clean Food
Good food hygiene by ensuring clean kitchens, appropriate storage and cooking of food and the appropriate use of clean utensils will reduce the risk of unnecessary infections and illnesses in the cancer fighter who has just finished traditional treatment which in many cases will have left their body more exposed due to a suppressed immune system. Particular care should be taken with cleanliness especially hands, surfaces and raw vegetables. Careful preparation and handling of raw meat, fish and eggs is always important. Always ensure food is stored at the right temperature and thoroughly cooked through to avoid serious complications such as listeria.

Supplements
Rightly or wrongly cancer fighters use dietary supplements. Sometimes it is due to direct advice from their cancer dietician other times it is because it has become the social norm. There are widespread anecdotal and research benefits of taking certain dietary supplements when fighting cancer.

The received wisdom is to not take more than the recommended daily intake for all vitamins and minerals where they exist. This however does not stop some cancer fighters taking more on the basis that the daily intake is for healthy adults not cancer fighters.

I will discuss vitamins in more detail later but in general terms the majority of evidence focuses on data for improved outcomes for vitamins A, C & E. However it is important to be aware in two clinical trials that for the precursor for vitamin A (beta-carotene) it was found to be dangerous to take more in cases of lung cancer and people that smoke. Other vitamins such as vitamin D and the vitamin Bs have been shown to be important parts of the diet of the cancer fighter. Key minerals such as selenium and calcium can play an important part in the diet of the cancer fighter too (especially those with colon cancer). The benefits and risks of using higher than daily recommended levels of antioxidants during cancer therapy is a hotly disputed area with doctors on both sides and no universally accepted agreement. It is as always best to consult your doctor about your specific situation but be aware that there appears to be as many for as against their use before and during treatment.

Many studies have shown that regular aerobic exercise can reduce anxiety and depression, improve mood, boost self-esteem, and reduce symptoms of fatigue. In general resistance and impact exercise can decrease the risk of osteoporosis in cancer fighters. Cancer fighters who are menopausal women and men with prostate cancer are at high risk for osteoporosis and so would probably benefit from exercises to increase bone strength.

Jobs to do

There is more detailed advice throughout the book but occasionally it is important to mention the obvious as sometimes as humans we overlook it as it is not always that stimulating. There are plenty of resources on the internet about diet and exercise but here are five to remind you of.

1. Get a referral to a registered dietician if possible.

2. Eat a healthy and balanced diet with whole grains, <u>no added sugar</u> and reduced meat intake (especially low for red and processed meats).

3. Eat <u>five or more</u> servings of a variety of vegetables and fruits each day.

4. Keep a healthy weight with limited saturated fats intake and do not do fad diets unless it includes lots of fruit and vegetables, oily fish and walnuts.

5. Do regular physical activity if able.

6. Drink plenty of water but not excessive amounts and only a little alcohol if you can!

Chapter 3: Mediterranean Diet & Super Herbs

It is widely accepted that a healthy diet is essential for good health and so I am not going to focus on all aspects of your diet but of course will recommend you refer to the web, a wealth of books and possibly a dietician for general and specific advice regarding this. Clearly there are many differing views on what constitutes a healthy diet but most involve plenty of unprocessed fruit and vegetables, limited amounts of red meat and processed food with low intakes of fat (especially saturated fats), salt and especially sugar. I want to focus on foods and supplements with widely researched benefits in cancer prevention and treatment.

From historical studies of human remains it would appear that cancer is more prevalent in modern times although this is slightly skewed as people tended to die early of other infections and diseases at an earlier age due to a lack of modern healthcare. It is also important to remember that those bodies found intact tend to be in burial chambers and therefore relate to the richer and therefore better fed and looked after people of the time. However it is fair to say that in the pre-smoking and pre-industrial age that cancers caused by pollutants were far less common and possibly diets with more emphasis on fruit and vegetables and low levels of meat intake were healthier.

It is now widely accepted that diet is an important part of health and well-being generally but especially heart disease. Heart disease is considered an inflammatory disease by many and a Mediterranean diet is considered good for reducing the amount of heart disease. Obviously a healthy circulatory system is of key importance in fighting cancer which is also considered an inflammatory or inflammatory-like disease. Like all biological systems that utilise chemicals for energy conversion there are often a large number of unwanted and potentially toxic by-products which are formed. These need to be processed and or removed as quickly as possible before they do any damage. A good circulatory system is required to achieve this whether by the lymphatic or blood system.

The benefits of a good Mediterranean diet and for that matter a good Japanese diet to both the cardio-vascular system and cancer prevention seem repeatedly linked. Just as with many things there is limited specific information and research about what exactly constitutes a Mediterranean diet. If you spoke to a Spaniard, Italian and Greek let alone a French or Portuguese chef they would happily and proudly argue for hours about the difference. I do not pretend to present the perfect answer but I will focus on the ones I feel are most interesting and relevant to cancer prevention and treatment. I must also point out that I am not a chef and have married into an Italian family so of course maybe biased or mad or both.

Antioxidants and vitamins will be discussed in later chapters in more detail but there is a lot of evidence that antioxidants and their activity are important in protecting against cell damage caused by other chemicals known as oxidants (free radicals). I think it is fair to say that most people would agree that the Mediterranean diet contains garlic, tomatoes, red wine and olive oil as key ingredients. Due to their importance I will talk about garlic and tomatoes in a lot of detail later. I will focus on red wine and olive oil first as these in particular contain some naturally occurring chemicals known as polyphenols. The polyphenols from fresh olives and red grapes have high levels of antioxidant activity. Luckily even after processing, the levels of resveratrol (a polyphenol) are quite high in red wine with other polyphenols also high in extra virgin olive oil.

It is well known that white blood cells (leucocytes) within blood are essential to help combat infection and are a vital part of your natural defence system. It is also widely accepted that the early stages of atherosclerosis, considered by most an inflammatory disease, is characterised by leucocytes sticking to the walls of arteries where they are obviously less likely to be of positive use to your body. Studies have shown both olive oil and red wine polyphenols reduce the overall stickiness of these leucocytes. They found that both the polyphenols from both olive oil and red wine were highly likely to be linked to a possible reduction in these plaques (fatty deposits) forming in arteries. These chemicals appear to have very many positive health impacts which help to limit the development of fatty deposits within arteries and general anti-inflammatory properties. One research study concluded in their findings that "better circulation may enable the body to be more effective generally and may help it in the fight against cancerous cells". This would seem to make sense but obviously is only a may be, however it is a very interesting study, which raises other questions such as maybe the anti-inflammatory properties these polyphenols exhibit may also have a direct impact on some cancers many consider an inflammatory disease.

On top of all the positive news regarding polyphenols and their anti-oxidant properties it has been found by scientists in the USA at Harvard University that polyphenols, which are chemicals made by plants extend the life of yeast cells by helping them to produce certain enzymes. "Yeast cells.....so what!" I hear you say, well the good news is that according to their research they also work to some degree on human cells. Even better news is that one of the widely researched polyphenols is resveratrol which is found in red wine. In 1997 it was shown that resveratrol was important during all periods of the cancer process: initiation, promotion and progression periods. So it appears that not only is red wine possibly good at reducing the likelihood of heart disease it also may be useful directly in the fight against cancer. These antioxidant and anticancer properties were found alongside an increase in the enzyme quinone reductase. This phase II enzyme is an enzyme which can reduce the impact of cancer causing chemicals (carcinogens). **This research and scientific discussion has shown and indicated that resveratrol is in fact highly active both in the reduction of incidence of cancerous activity and the reduction of cancerous activity and progression, so potentially useful as a complimentary treatment**.

If you think this area is an interesting bit of research, but is it really all that, I can tell you it is certainly big business and that back in 2007 a very serious player in the phytochemical industry, Xenomis signed an exclusive licensing agreement with Harvard Medical School for the development of polyphenol products specifically focussed on this research area which commits them to investing several million dollars. Although this could of course just mean it is likely to be profitable, most companies do not knowingly invest large sums of money in areas they feel are not likely to be worthwhile and proven in the long term.

Unfortunately no scientists or doctors have said that the more red wine you drink the better you get but who is to say a little bit of what you like regularly does not help you in the fight against your cancer. Clearly no scientific paper is going to recommend drinking red wine to excess but I feel it is useful information which can be incorporated into your daily health regime and cancer treatment in a mature and grown-up way.

My personal recommendations assume you have informed your doctor of your intentions and sought their advice regarding any negative health effects or interactions with your formal medical/surgical treatment.

But I recommend a glass of the best red wine and half a shot glass of the best virgin olive oil you can afford every day. Red wine as a rule seems to have higher levels of resveratrol, but if you do not drink red wine, then buy a quality pure red grape juice ideally with as little additives as possible. The resveratrol appears in the highest concentration within the red grape skins compared to white grapes I am afraid to say for you white wine lovers. It is noted that cranberries and blueberries also have levels present in their juice however to a lesser degree.

Dietary Fats and Cholesterol
People's fat intake has been the pre-occupation of the late twentieth century and the beginning of this one for the developed countries. The fat we eat can be subdivided into three major types of fatty acid: saturated, monounsaturated and polyunsaturated fatty acid. The big two polyunsaturated fatty acids are omega-3 and omega-6. There are two polyunsaturated fatty acids that can't be produced by the human body and these are linoleic acid (omega-6 family) and linolenic acid (omega-3 family). They must be eaten and so are known as essential fatty acids. Linoleic acid (omega-6) is present in most vegetable seeds oils and is the main polyunsaturated fatty acid in the Western diet.

The omega-3 fatty acids include linolenic acid and its chemical products eicosapentaenoic acid and docosahexaenoic acid. The main food sources of these omega-3 fatty acids are flaxseeds, margarine, fish oils and shellfish.

There are many research studies including laboratory and human studies which show a low fat diet (e.g. less than 20% of diet) has a significant positive effect in the fight against cancer both in the occurrence and treatment of cancers.

It is believed that high-fat diets may influence cancers especially prostate cancer through their complex link with testosterone and sex hormones. Levels of testosterone have been seen to decrease with a reduction in fat intake.

It is equally important to be aware that also more specific aspects of fat intake like the percentage split between saturated, monounsaturated, and polyunsaturated fats have been studied. Interestingly there are many quality studies which show a significant protective benefit of omega-3 fatty acids and the opposite for omega-6 fatty acids which show increased cancer risk. In simple terms it would appear the good fat for fighting cancer is omega-3 fatty acids and the bad fat is the omega-6 fatty acids. These studies help to confirm the belief that populations with a high fish (oil) intake tend to have less cancer than those that don't when you assume all other variables are equal.

In a large research study of over 6,000 Swedish men lasting over 30 years, it was found that men who ate no fish had a 200 to 300% increased chance of prostate cancer than men who ate fish regularly.

Decreasing fat intake overall also helps reduce the risk of cardiovascular disease, which is another example of a health benefit for the heart being also a health benefit to the cancer fighter.

Many detailed studies have shown that diets high in saturated and hydrogenated fats lead to increased occurrence of inflammatory conditions, however the opposite is true for diets which are high in unsaturated fats such as the so-called Mediterranean diet. These diets that are high in unsaturated fats can help reduce inflammation. A Mediterranean diet emphasizes olive oil, fruits and vegetables, nuts, beans, fish, whole grains, and small consumption of alcohol especially red wine. Most of these foods are important sources of fatty acids that are involved in inflammatory processes. Higher intakes of the omega-3 fatty acids (i.e., alpha-linolenic acid (ALA), eicosapentaenoic acid (EPA), and docosahexaenoic acid (DHA)) have been generally associated with decreased incidence of inflammation. Dietary sources rich in ALA include flaxseeds and their oil, walnuts and their oil, and canola oil. EPA and DHA are found in oily fish and fish oils. The ratio of omega-6 to omega-3 fatty acids in the typical Western diet is about 18:1, yet it is estimated that humans before industrialization had a diet with an omega-6 to omega-3 fatty acid ratio of about 1:1. It is therefore believed that by reducing the actual intake ratio to be closer to 1:1 will help reduce the number and degree of many inflammatory conditions observed in Western societies (see oxidative stress chapters for more information).

Low cholesterol diets are widely advised for people suffering from cardio-vascular disease but there is significant evidence that lower cholesterol levels help reduce inflammation throughout the body. An interesting study in America found that a very high cholesterol diet over a month period increased the levels of two inflammatory markers in people significantly, whereas fatter people who had a low cholesterol diet over a similar period had lower levels of inflammatory markers.

Population studies seem to indicate that the daily consumption of extra-virgin olive oil lowers the incidence of certain types of cancer, in particular bladder cancer. Recent evaluation of the antiproliferative activity in bladder cancers of the polyphenols present in extra-virgin olive oil on bladder cancer seem to clarify the biological mechanisms that trigger cell death. Even more interesting is that a recent study showed low doses of extra-virgin olive oil when taken in conjunction with 2 cancer drugs (paclitaxel and mitomycin) enhanced their effectiveness in controlling cancer growth. Their results showed that extra-virgin olive oil significantly stopped the proliferation of the cancer in a linear fashion. The cancer drug, mitomycin showed a reduction in its cytotoxic side effects when taken with extra-virgin olive oil, whilst the cancer drug, paclitaxel and extra-virgin olive oil strongly increased cell death of cancer cells.

Extra virgin olive oil is preferred as it comes from the first pressing of the olives without any additives or refining process and thus contains high levels of phenolic compounds. In particular two main phenolic compounds appear important oleuropein aglycone and decarboxymethyl oleuropein aglycone seem to interfere with the production of growth factor-β which plays an important role in cancer and tissue degeneration. It is interesting that many natural anti-inflammatory foodstuffs in the diet are also highly effective at clearing the body of parasitic worms these foodstuffs are known as natural anthelmintic and are readily available such as cloves, garlic and pineapple. Pineapples are so important that they will be covered in more detail later.

Phytoestrogens

Phytoestrogens are naturally occurring plant compounds that are classified as flavones, isoflavones, and lignans. These compounds display estrogen-like activity because as chemicals their structure is similar to the body's own oestrogen. It is thought often that this structural similarity is what may be protective for prostate cancer by reducing the impact of testosterone. Isoflavones like genistein interfere with 5alpha-reductase activity. The 5alpha-reductase enzyme enables the conversion of testosterone into its more dihydrotestosterone active form. This active form is known to stimulate the growth of prostate gland.

Genistein has been shown to inhibit the growth of prostate cancer cells in vitro. By using human prostate LNCaP tumor cells, physiologic concentrations of genistein (< 20 µmol/L) reduced the number of viable cells in a dose-dependent manner. This concentration also decreased PSA mRNA expression a commonly used measure (although a little blunt) in prostate cancer treatment. Higher concentrations of genistein (> 20 µmol/L) also induced apoptosis.

By culturing human prostate cancer cells with genistein, Geller and his fellow researchers found that tissue conversion into prostate cancer tissue was significantly reduced. Independent of the effects on cell growth, isoflavones have also been shown to inhibit the metastatic activity of prostate cancer cells. Another mechanism of action could be the effect of isoflavones on angiogenesis (formation of new blood vessels to feed new/cancer cells). It has been seen that high concentrations of genistein inhibit angiogenesis, a process necessary for tumour growth and so that genistein may also be useful in the fight against cancer.

Animal models again provide the most provocative data. With use of so-called Lobund-Wistar rats, which are inherently predisposed to develop spontaneous prostate tumours, animals receiving a high-isoflavone diet had a significantly reduced incidence of prostate cancer compared with rats receiving a low-isoflavone diet. In a different model, growth of LNCaP prostate cancer cells transplanted into nude mice was inhibited by soy. However, when these tumors became palpable, there was no longer any difference in growth rates between the treatment groups. This suggests that soy probably exerts its beneficial effect during the early stages of tumour development and that the effect on established palpable tumours may be more limited.

Soy has been found to reduce tumour angiogenesis and enhance apoptosis in mice with tumours. Also insulin growth factor-1 levels were significantly lower in mice fed a high-soy diet than a control group. It is therefore possible that the insulin growth factor-1 may be important to consider when researching the process of angiogenesis. This links nicely to the already noted impact of excess sugar (glucose) in tumour growth. Interestingly when rats were fed genistein their androgen receptors were dampened down in a linear fashion related to the intake of genistein which could have a significant role to play in prostrate cancers.

In a review of soy products impact on tumours in 31 animal studies it was found that in 23 there was a reduction in tumour growth. Very few specific human studies have taken place to review the effects of phytoestrogens.

A large study in the USA of more than 12,000 men found that regular drinking of soy milk led to a massive risk reduction of 70% in the incidence of prostate cancer. Such a large study should not be overlooked as a potential guide in the fight against prostate cancer. However this study was of Seventh-Day Adventist males only and so it should be remembered that such a study leads to other potentially confounding factors due to their lifestyle and general diet differences. This being understood 70% is still a large difference in this population and so is worthy of consideration. Other smaller but randomized, placebo-controlled studies involving the intake of soy protein and its effect on prostate cancer have shown similar positive responses with many studies still active in this area.

It is proving to be useful in men who even after radical surgery are having high levels of Prostate Specific Antigen (PSA). This unfortunately negative and common situation of even after surgery is widely known as PSA failure. This is because high PSA levels mean an increased likelihood of cancer occurring again. It is now more widely accepted for prostate cancer that soy protein and other phytoestrogens are highly beneficial in terms of avoidance and reducing re-occurrence.

Herbs

It appears that many, if not most, herbs apart from making food taste better also have medicinal benefits including impacting on cancer growth. The commonly used herbs mint, rosemary, sage, oregano and thyme have been shown to have hormonal impacts similar to oestrogen reducing testosterone levels which is linked to cancer growth. There is a need to review their potency and effect on a wide range of cancers apart from testosterone-affected tumours but in small doses they are not going to do any major harm but have the potential for benefit outweighing their obvious flavouring benefits. They contain complex chemicals such as polyphenols, flavones and terpenoids which can impact the body's metabolism in complex ways. Ground Cloves & Saffron these 2 spices have been traded across the world for not just hundreds but thousands of years and have rightly been valued highly and at different times in history have been valued higher than gold. Cloves originated in a few Indonesian islands which became known as the Spice Islands but were traded for their taste and curative powers in the Middle East and Europe long ago. Cloves have long been one of the most valued spices.

The herbs and spices greatly valued by the Great Empires and civilized worlds are also those which have not only flavour but significant health benefits such as **Parsley, Cloves, saffron, nutmeg and pepper.**

Parsley is a wonder food which is often overlooked. **Parsley** contains a multitude of chemicals which can be very helpful in your fight against cancer. There are essential oils such as myristicin, limonene, eugenol, and alpha-thujene. And there are important flavonoids such as apiin, apigenin, crisoeriol, and luteolin. Myristicin is also found in **nutmeg** in large amounts has the ability to stop some cancers forming and also acts as an activator to glutathione-S-transferase formation. Myristicin has also been found to work extremely well at ensuring the liver's health and function

Saffron is another wonder food which is often overlooked due to its price, which demonstrates its true value as more than just a food flavouring. It contains a wide range of chemicals including many carotenoids such as lycopene and has been the subject of widespread research for its cancer fighting properties both in terms of prevention of re-occurrence and as part of a treatment regime. It has been repeatedly shown to be beneficial in animal and human test-tube cell tests.

Cloves
Cloves are packed with manganese and also a wide range of exciting chemicals including Caryophyllene which has anti-inflammatory properties also present in Black Pepper, Basil, Cinnamon, Oregano, Rosemary & Hops. Cloves due to their chemical contents also have antiseptic and painkilling properties which have been used for centuries. Cloves also contain polyphenols like gallotannic acid, terpenoids like oleanolic acid (also in garlic) and flavonoids like

kaempferol (also in onions, capers & tea) which have been noted for their anti-inflammatory and anti-cancer properties. Cloves also contain a chemical called Eugenol which is very powerful and also toxic if too much is taken. Anybody who has accidentally swallowed a clove whilst eating a curry will testify that the body reacts to it quite significantly and that cloves need to be treated with some respect. Ground cloves provide the most manganese with approximately 30mg present in 100 grams of cloves which is considered to be 1502% of the RDA. Saffron is estimated to contain high levels of Manganese as well when compared to most other foodstuffs which are approximately half the amount of Cloves weight for weight.

It is important to be aware that clove oil although used for many centuries for painful teeth and gums is in fact highly concentrated and is not to be drunk. Clove oil and especially eugenol is very powerful and toxic and should not be taken directly by mouth without significant dilution and definitely not regularly.

Cloves have a complex biochemistry which consists of a mix of eugenol, acids, tannins, triterpenoids and flavonoids. Many of these such as Kaempferol appear to have significant impacts on different cancers impeding their growth and proliferation whilst also stimulating cancer cell death.

Cloves have potent antioxidant and antimicrobial properties which further enhance their use medically. Cloves we traditionally associate for cooking come from the clove tree (Syzygium aromaticum) which grows up to approximately 12 metres tall. They are originally from the Maluku islands in east Indonesia. Nowadays, the tree is farmed widely around the world with Indonesia, India, Malaysia, Sri Lanka, Madagascar and Tanzania being significant producers of cloves. In

Brazil clove is farmed with nearly 8,000 hectares of land used and 2,500 tons per year produced. For hundreds of years this spice has been traded for medicinal and culinary uses. The tree is often cultivated in coastal areas. The production of the flower buds, which is the part used for cooking begins after 4 years. Flower buds are collected before flowering.

Cloves contain many phenolic compounds such as flavonoids, hidroxibenzoic acids, hidroxicinamic acids and hidroxiphenyl propens. Eugenol is the main bioactive compound of clove and plays a significant role in cloves anti-cancer properties. Eugenol can interfere with several cell-signalling pathways, especially the nuclear factor kappa B (NFkB). This factor is activated by free radicals and results in the stimulation of genes that suppress apoptosis and induce cellular transformation, proliferation, invasion and even metastasis.

Eugenol is very powerful as it has anti-oxidative and cytotoxic properties as well as being able to damage DNA. Its abilities have been tested in a study with regard to its ability to interfere with the damaging effects of hydrogen peroxide (a potentially damaging oxidant) on DNA of different types of cancerous human cells including malignant liver cells, malignant colon cells and healthy fibroblast cells. The study showed that eugenol was strongly anti-oxidative and also cytotoxic, whilst also damaging to DNA in the fibroblast cells, however based on several long term cancer studies eugenol is not considered carcinogenic to rats. Further study has shown that eugenol can suppress the growth of the melanomas, decrease the size of tumours and resist melanoma invasion of tissue and metastasis. Eugenol achieves this impact on melanomas by the reduction and interference of two transition factors (E2F group of genes).

Eugenol is a complex chemical that at low concentrations acts as an antioxidant but paradoxically acts as an oxidant stimulator at high concentrations. Research suggests that eugenol inhibits the enzyme MMP-9 which is related to metastasis in human fibrosarcoma cells. This research indicates that eugenol could be used for prevention of metastasis that is related to oxidative stress.

Of the phenolic acids present in cloves, gallic acid and its derivatives are the compounds also found in high concentrations. Other powerful phenolic acids found in smaller concentrations are the caffeic, ferulic, elagic and salicylic acids. The key flavonoids but significantly lower concentrations are kaempferol are quercetin. Other important compounds found in cloves are α-humulen, β-pinene, limonene, farnesol, benzaldehyde, 2-heptanone and ethyl hexanoate.

Cloves are up there as one of the top spices with the highest polyphenol and antioxidant content according to the United States Department of Agriculture. The USDA created a database with the polyphenol content and antioxidant activity of different kind of foods. The database shows that spices are the type of food with the higher polyphenol content. After spices the other foods with high polyphenols are fruits, seeds and vegetables.

The antioxidant activity of clove was reviewed using in vitro models and direct comparison methods. The research showed that the antioxidant activity of clove is similar in strength to butylated hydroxytoluene which is a powerful synthetic antioxidant historically used as food preservative. The powerful antioxidant activity appears to be related to eugenol's active scavenging of free radicals, hydrogen peroxide and superoxide. Studies show consistently that cloves' polyphenols are complex in their antioxidant behaviour. These polyphenols can act as reducing agents, hydrogen atom donors, and single oxygen scavengers.

The eugenol molecule has an interesting structure of the carbon atoms with an aromatic ring which absorbs light in a similar way to the molecule of resveratrol which is another important antioxidant with research ongoing with regards to cancer care.

The anti-bacterial and anti-fungal properties of cloves have been demonstrated against several different bacteria and fungi. The water-diluted extract of cloves at 3% concentration has controlled colonies of the following bacteria Escherichia coli (E. coli), Listeria monocitogenes, Staphylococcus aureus and Bacillus cereus and with effects present even at lower concentrations.

Eugenol can inhibit the growth of at least 31 different strains of Helicobacter pylori. Eugenol has been seen to be more potent that amoxicillin in fighting this bacteria and without developing resistance. This bacterium is very aggressive once it has the right conditions and has been shown to be responsible for gastric ulcers and much study continues regarding its potential for causing gastric cancer and others. The bacteria and the toxins it produces induce a local inflammatory response leading to increased concentration of inflammation-associated signalling molecules, such as Tumour Necrosis Factor Alpha and InterLeukin 6. Continued high levels of these have been linked to increased opportunity for cancer to develop.

The anti-fungal activity of clove oil in different strains of fungi (e.g. Microsporum gypseum, Trichophytum rubrum, Pseudomonas aeruginosa & Aspergillus sp.) was seen to be due to lysis of the spores and micelles. Further study showed that eugenol was the main chemical responsible for the anti-fungal activity. After cancer chemotherapy many people find their immune system is compromised and they are more liable to Candida infections such as Thrush and luckily dilute clove oil has anti-candidal activity.

The antiviral activity of cloves appears to interfere with viral DNA synthesis of some important viruses such as herpes simplex virus type 1 (HSV-1).

The use of clove as an analgesic has occurred probably since their use as a spice. Most commonly it is still used for mild toothache, joint pain and for colic-like pain. It appears that this action is due to the stimulation of calcium and chloride channels in neural cells. It is interesting that other studies consider that the analgesic effect of cloves is due to the action as capsaicin agonist. Later we will see that capsaicin is also of interest in the fight against cancer.

Garlic

Again the link between the medicinal benefit and the ancient culinary use of certain herbs and spices is present in garlic. Garlic has long been used for its medicinal properties and more recently its role in cancer prevention and reduction. There is significant use of garlic in the majority of Mediterranean diets and much research to support garlic's strong anti-cancer benefits. These anti-cancer benefits from garlic could come from its bactericidal properties or from its ability to block angiogenesis and cell proliferation whilst inducing apoptosis commonly called cell death in cancer cells.

Of particular interest in the treatment of prostate cancer have been lab studies that show garlic interferes with growth of androgen-dependent prostate cancer cells. In keeping with many other substances that impact cancer cells it is possible that garlic may stimulate P450 enzymes, which are important for toxin metabolism. From recent studies it appears that fresh garlic seems to exert a greater influence than tablet, processed or dried garlic.

Many large studies across the world from China to Europe looking at cause, type and prognosis of cancer treatment have shown a definite association between high garlic consumption and reduced risk of many cancers, including cancers of the gastric tract, pancreas and breast. The results from European Prospective Investigation into Cancer and Nutrition (EPIC) are also broadly in agreement with the benefits of fresh garlic in cancer prevention. This is a massive, long term study, which is analysing male and female data from 10 different countries. Several population studies conducted in China focussed on garlic consumption and cancer risk. One key placebo-controlled clinical study of interest was of 5,000 Chinese men and women at high risk for stomach cancer. The study reviewed the impact of taking a combination of 200mg of garlic extract and 100 micrograms selenium every other day and with another group taking a daily placebo for 5 years. The garlic extract and selenium group had a reduced risk of over 30% for all cancers and for stomach cancer in particular they had a reduced risk of over 50% compared to the placebo group.

One study showed that frequent consumption of garlic and various types of onions was linked with reduced risk of stomach cancers. A practically linear relationship was found with more garlic eaten leading to greater reduction in risk of stomach, colon and prostate cancer. One American study found that pancreatic cancer risk was over 50% less in people who ate larger amounts of garlic compared with those who didn't. One French study found that breast cancer risk was significantly reduced in people who ate larger amounts of garlic compared with those who didn't.

There is a wealth of evidence that garlic inhibits angiogenesis, that is to say it interferes with production of a blood supply to tumours. Garlic is agreed to offer protection against the likelihood of gastric and colon cancers. In the famous female study in Iowa of over 41,000 women reviewing over 120 different types of food, garlic showed a major benefit in women having one or more servings of fresh garlic a week. These women had over 35% less colon cancer and the results are in keeping with the Chinese study in 1998 which showed reduced cancers in people having regular fresh garlic. Excess cooking such as frying or roasting seems to be much less effective. Once again it appears that much of garlic's health benefit appears to be derived from its antioxidant as well as its bactericidal, anti-fungal, anti-microbial and anti-viral properties.

Fungi, Bacteria and other microbes have multiple purposes within the eco-system that is the human body with so-called good and bad relationships (i.e. symbiotic and parasitic) with them. The parasitic types are a drain on the body in terms of using up valuable resources such as vitamins, especially Vitamin Bs that play key roles in DNA duplication and the immune response. In addition these microbes can produce dangerous toxins.

There are many active chemicals in garlic but it appears that allicin plays an important role. The well-known smell of garlic comes from the organosulphur chemical, allicin. In addition to the allicin, garlic also contains the following chemicals, arginine, flavonoids and selenium, which can convey health benefits and also impact on cancer prevention and growth.

One small simple study showed that the application of liquid garlic extract to some skin cancers may be beneficial. In the study of 21 people with basal cell carcinoma, applying the extract to the skin for 1 month reduced the size of 17 tumours significantly.

The National Cancer Institute of the USA which is known for its conservative approach doesn't suggest any dietary supplements as useful for the prevention of cancer due to what it feels is a lack of scientific evidence, but it does state that garlic like many other plants has anticancer potential. The studies completed use different extraction techniques and concentrations of garlic, so it is hard to collate the evidence to date in a more solid or meaningful way. This means that recommending amounts or particular extracts is difficult. Apart from the well-known smell of garlic after eating both on breath and sweat, large quantities of garlic can cause vomiting and diarrhoea. Some studies indicate that garlic can in fact lower blood sugar levels and increase insulin. The link between high blood sugar levels and cancer growth and proliferation is widely accepted as an extenuating factor and so garlic's impact on reducing sugar levels may further explain how garlic interferes with cancer. Generally this impact is a useful thing, but for diabetics managing their diabetes with insulin it is an important side effect to be aware of. Equally garlic can act as a natural blood thinner so should be taken in consultation with your oncologist, doctor or dietician.

Garlic contains a range of sulphur-based chemicals, which are believed to play a significant role in garlic's health benefits including potential to prevent and treat cancer and heart disease. The sulphur-based chemicals include glutamylcysteines and cysteine sulfoxides. Allylcysteine sulfoxide (alliin) makes up approximately 80% of the cysteine sulfoxides in garlic. When raw garlic cloves are crushed, chopped, or chewed, the enzyme, alliinase is activated. This enzyme is a significant part of a cascade of different reactions; some of these actually result in sulphenic acids and thiosulphinates. One key thiosulphinate is allicin which also leads to other important chemicals. Allicin and its derived chemicals are absorbed by the body following ingestion, however their biological impacts are poorly understood. Allicin and allicin-derived chemicals, including ajoene, diallylsufides and vinyldithiins appear to be used by the body as they have never been detected in human blood and urine, or stool after ingestion.

Garlic and its associated allicin products have been shown to decrease the production of cholesterol by liver cells. In addition to this potential health benefit garlic and its associated allicin products have also shown the ability to limit blood clotting be interfering with platelet aggregation and to reduce the activity of the inflammatory enzymes, cyclooxygenase and lipoxygenase. More recently, organosulphur chemicals have been found in lab studies to decrease the production of inflammatory signalling molecules in white blood cells and human blood. A number of these chemicals also have significant antioxidant activity and that some even appear to stimulate glutathione production. Glutathione is an important antioxidant present inside cells which helps prevent oxidative damage to DNA.

Cancers are primarily a consequence of unregulated cell division. The cell cycle is tightly regulated in normal cells to ensure correct DNA replication prior to cell division. When there is significant oxidative damage to DNA, the cell cycle can be stopped to allow for DNA repair or actively altered towards cell death (apoptosis). Apoptosis is a normal cell process for the self-destruction of cells that have DNA damage or no longer required. Precancerous and cancerous cells are often resistant to the normal cell signals that induce cell cycle arrest and apoptosis. The organosulphur chemicals from garlic including allicin and ajoene can induce apoptosis when added to various cancer cells in the lab. In animal studies aqueous garlic extract taken orally can enhance apoptosis in oral cancers in particular.

Even though garlic and its associated compounds have been found to reduce the development of oral, gastric, colon, cervical, breast, prostate and skin cancers in animal studies there is still limited evidence in human studies. Not only has garlic been seen to have effects on cardio-vascular disease by appearing to inhibit platelet aggregation and reduce cholesterol but also is strongly anti-bactericidal and anti-fungal. It is known that some bacterial and fungal infections can increase the incidence of cancer. For example Infection with some strains of Helicobacter pylori bacteria markedly increases the risk of gastric cancer. It is clear that garlic and its extracts perform best when fresh and not extensively processed or cooked. This is understood to be because the enzyme alliinase can be denatured by heat. It has become clear that once crushed or chopped the alliinase is activated and should be left to continue to work for approximately ten minutes before eating or very lightly cooking on a low heat. Much of the powdered garlic or dried supplements contain less active ingredients and so fresh is best followed by liquid "fresh" extracts and finally by dried garlic. Garlic preparations have been found to stop the growth of H. pylori in the lab, however this yet to be proved in humans beyond doubt.

Green tea

Green tea although not a herb as such is packed with organic chemicals, which appear to be highly active and may impact cancers significantly. Green tea is a good source of epicatechin flavonoids and tea generally are a rich source of flavonoids with green tea containing the most. Green tea is made by steaming or frying tea leaves and then drying them. It is mainly drunk in China and Japan, where it has been used for medicinal purposes for more than 5,000 years. In recent years it is more widely drunk in the West as the world's populations move and become more integrated. Green tea contains a number of phytochemicals, of which the polyphenols are the most common. The main polyphenol is epigallocatechin gallate (EGCG), which has been extensively studied in cell and animal studies. EGCG is the single most studied catechin regarding health benefits as it the major flavonoid present in green tea. It represents up to 75% of all flavonoid content in green tea.

All tea contains many active antioxidant polyphenols. Black tea, green tea and oolong teas have antioxidant properties. All three varieties come from the same plant Camellia sinenis. Contrary to popular belief black tea do contain some antioxidants, but by far the most potent source is green tea (jasmine tea) which contains the antioxidant catechin. Black tea has only about 10 per cent as many antioxidants as green tea. Oolong tea has more antioxidants than black tea and by far the winner is green tea (jasmine tea). This is because some of the antioxidants are destroyed, when green tea is turned into black tea. Many of the catechins are oxidized during black tea production and converted to thearubigins with theaflavins making up the minority key content of flavonoids. Other even lower content flavonoids in tea are kaempferol, myricetin, quercetin, apigenin and luteolin.

Interestingly EGCG has been seen to induce apoptosis in human prostate and other cancer cells. In fact by injecting green tea extracts into mice that had cancers the tumours have been seen to stop growing and also shrink rather than the controls expected growth. The link was so clear that when the green tea injections were stopped the tumours started to grow again. This amazing link was repeatable and was equally noted when EGCG was injected. Even taking green tea extracts by mouth was noted to have an effect as well as the complete arrest of further metastases. This is only for prostate cancers in mice but if animal studies have any validity then this is a truly exciting area of potential cancer research and treatment. There are few if any large human studies showing significant benefits and so this does need to be considered, however there are equally few if any large human studies showing no benefits.

Jobs to do

1. Have a glass of red wine per day
2. Have a half a shot glass of extra virgin olive oil per day
3. Have 4 cups of green tea per day
4. Buy cloves and garlic to put in meals where possible or grind up and have a ½ teaspoon of each per day
5. Buy fresh herbs such as parsley, saffron, cloves rosemary, mint and sage for daily meals
6. Reduce meat especially red meat and fat intake
7. Have oily fish such as sardines three times per week
8. Buy more nuts, flaxseed and fruit generally (not grapefruit)
9. Buy soy milk and soy protein

Chapter 4: Vitamin A, C, D, E & Selenium

This is for your information only but there is such little agreement that I would not advised higher levels than the Recommended Daily Allowance.

Vitamin A is an essential (the human body does not make it) vitamin that is well known for its impact on the eye and that as children many of us were told to eat lots of carrots to help us see in the dark. Vitamin A and its precursors are found in a range of foodstuffs particularly liver, fish and milk products.

Isomers (chemicals closely related to retinoic acid) of Vitamin A have been seen to act as hormones that affect gene expression and transcription. This hormone-like action impacts on the production of key proteins which are involved in important cell physiological processes. Vitamin A isomers are also seen to interact with Vitamin D and thyroid and growth hormones, which also play important roles in metabolic processes. It is therefore fairly easy to see that Vitamin A plays an important role in cell physiology, growth and differentiation and thus potentially cancer.

The ability of retinoic acid (vitamin A) to inhibit cancer growth is well known and widely accepted, although exactly how it works is not fully understood. This link between vitamin A and cancer was noted in 1926 when rats that were fed a diet with no vitamin A suffered from cancer of the gut. Vitamin A fights cancer it seems by reducing the production of DNA in cancer cells and slowing down cancer growth even very aggressive cancers such as leukaemia. Recently there has been some media interpretation of some research which led to people believing that Vitamin A could lead to increased cancer growth. This stems from the fact that beta-carotene yielded conflicting results regarding its benefits or negative impact on prostate cancer. This has been during test-tube research only on prostate cancer cells and does not appear to be duplicated in animal research due to the fact that the beta-carotene is a pre-cursor to Vitamin A and so is converted to Vitamin A before it can help fight cancer growth. The prostate gland and cancer seem by their biochemical nature to be at significant risk to oxidative stress and related DNA damage caused by ROS. It is believed that the prostrate is at most risk due to its high level of activity and cell growth generally also linked to its general susceptibility to inflammation. It appears from larger studies that it depends on what your initial body levels of Vitamin A are before increased intake is started and the effect. In a large scale cancer prevention study of 29,000 male smokers taking Vitamin E & Beta-Carotene supplements there was an increased risk (18%) of lung cancer for those smoking men taking the supplements over those not. This is unfortunate because although Vitamin A is involved in a range of metabolic reactions relating to cell growth it is in fact a highly utilized chemical in the fight against cancer and blindness especially night blindness. Liver & carrots contain high levels of carotenoids which can be converted into vitamin A, which is why as children rather simplistically many of us were told to eat lots of carrots to help us see in the dark. Carrots contain beta-carotene, which is the pigment responsible for making carrots orange. Beta-carotene is found concentrated in deep orange and green vegetables (the green chlorophyll covers up the orange pigment). Beta-carotene is an antioxidant that has been much discussed in connection with lung cancer rates. The evidence is conflicting; with one study showing an increase in risk, but further research is being done to see if it has a protective effect.

Carotenoids are complex compounds made up of many, many hundreds of naturally occurring pigments. The human body cannot create carotenoids by adding different foodstuffs together and so these chemicals must be eaten in the first place to be used by the body. Beta-carotene and lycopene are the main eaten carotenoids, however other carotenoids are present in fair amounts in fruits and vegetables. Carotenoids are the pigment compounds that give many fruits and vegetables their red, orange and yellow colour Carotenoids are the red, orange and yellow plant pigments that give fruits and vegetables their vivid colours. All fruits and vegetables contain varying concentrations of carotenoids, but their colours are often covered up by green chlorophyll contained in the plant. Carotenoids are plant based antioxidants. They include beta carotene, lutein and lycopene.

Many carotenoids, like beta-carotene, are precursors to Vitamin A in that they can be biochemically changed to vitamin A. It is also true though that the human body cannot change lycopene into Vitamin A. Lycopene is so important that it has been discussed in some detail already in Chapter 6. It is widely thought that carotenoids are highly important chemical complexes which help protect the body from the damage caused by ROS using their antioxidant properties. There is also mounting research which suggests that carotenoids also are directly involved in cell processes such as differentiation and growth which are directly related to cancer occurrence and growth.

Retinoic acid is an oxidised form of retinol, vitamin A. Retinoic acid control is important as it acts as a growth factor for cells especially epithelial cells. Although intuitively you would consider a growth factor not a useful thing for fighting cancer. It appears that it helps regulate regular normal growth and not cancerous growth thereby leading some cancers to shrink as normal service is resumed. That is normal growth takes over with normal cell death which is an essential part of fighting cancer. So increase vitamin A levels seems to lead to healthy cell changes, which is why it is used by many doctors around the world in cancer treatments. Clearly Vitamin A is not a wonder drug but should be considered an important part of your arsenal in your fight against cancer. It is important to remember that many Vitamins work well together for example it has been found that when providing both vitamin A and vitamin C to human breast cancer cells the reduction in cancer growth is significant in comparison to single Vitamin or no provision. It is not just gut, breast and prostate cancer that have found positive benefits from increased Vitamin A levels but a wide range of cancers. Vitamin A in doses higher than the recommended daily allowance have not been shown cause major problems for short duration but obviously as with all intake particular care should be taken if you are pregnant but a lack of vitamin A during pregnancy and infancy can cause significant birth defects like a weakened immune system, and blindness.

The National Institute of Health in the USA which is known for its reserve in statements states that there appears an association between diets rich in beta-carotene and vitamin A and a lower risk of many types of cancer. A higher intake of green and yellow vegetables or other food sources of beta carotene and/or vitamin A may decrease the risk of stomach and lung cancer.

Vitamin A (general term to include all isomers, pre- and post-cursors) is important in helping to maintain healthy skin and mucosa and thus in maintaining your immune system. Vitamin A is necessary to maintain the development of white blood cells, which not only are important for your immune system and so also play an important part in your body's inflammatory response as explained in more detail in the oxidative stress chapter. Vitamin A excesses and deficiencies are well known to cause serious birth and growth defects. Vitamin A is also involved in red blood cells growth and utilization of iron. Such that it is widely advised if anaemic that not only iron but also Vitamin A be taken to aid recovery. Vitamin A also has a complex relationship with zinc which if deficient also leads to poor utilization of Vitamin A.

Interestingly there have been varying results both positive and negative published in scientific journals regarding its importance in fighting a range of cancers. Often with test-tube tests (in vitro) on live cells showing benefits which are not duplicated in animal/human (in vivo) studies. However a large longitudinal study in the USA involving ten and a half thousand men showed no increased prostate cancer risk for those taking additional Vitamin A supplements.

There have been some noted benefits in sufferers of acute leukaemia but this is by no means extensive improvement across the majority. Whilst there has been serious problems noted in lung cancer sufferers who have taken increased levels of Vitamin A especially among those caused by environmental factors such as smoking. Many big studies have shown little major benefit for the majority of cancers and so it is best not to stray from the recommended daily amounts. High potency vitamin A supplements should not be used without medical supervision due to the risk of toxicity.

Vitamin C

Vitamin C is well documented as a key antioxidant and probably the most well-known. The body needs Vitamin C as an essential nutrient and uses it to manage oxidative damage by ROS. It is involved in many important processes within the body. Its antioxidant properties have linked it to a wide range of treatments for a range of inflammatory conditions particularly cardiovascular disease and cancer. It is heavily linked to our immune system with its ability to impact on the production of cytokines, lymphocytes and cell adhesion molecules and for many years people have increased their Vitamin C intake either with orange juice or supplements during colds to help their bodies' immune systems.

Vitamin C has a long history of being used as an anti-cancer treatment with many studies showing that Vitamin C is very useful in the fight against cancer both directly and as a means of minimising the deleterious impacts of radio and chemotherapy. It has been given orally and by injection to cancer patients. Vitamin C can be directly toxic to cancer cells specifically due to their low levels of the enzyme Catalase when compared to normal healthy cells which generally have significantly larger amounts of this antioxidant enzyme. The properties of Vitamin C can then be focused on the cancer cells as the normal cells manage the hydrogen peroxide production with their catalase. Due to cancer cells high levels of activity they need high levels of glucose and to obtain this quickly enough the cancer cells need more openness to glucose which luckily means they are also more open to Vitamin C which act destructively on the cancerous cells. The concentration levels for the best effect of Vitamin C on cancerous cells are in fact obtained by intravenous injection. It is not advisable to try this yourself as medical considerations need to be accounted for as some cancers can bleed after being treated with high dose vitamin C. Many good studies focusing on Vitamin C and its fight against cancer have not shown large changes in success for oral supplementation with Vitamin C. However many opposing researchers argue, that although they were good studies in their opinion insufficiently large amounts of Vitamin C were taken and also other combination effects were not considered. High levels of Vitamin C can be taken by mouth and have been seen to be highly beneficial in the fight against cancer but not significantly for everyone and the impact is definitely less effective in those cases than intravenously delivered Vitamin C.

Vitamin C (ascorbic acid) is widely found in citrus fruits and raw leafy vegetables. It is an essential water-soluble vitamin as the human body is unable to make it. **Vitamin C has a wide range of physiologic and metabolic functions. It is a well-known antioxidant which offers protection from damage caused by oxidants.**

Vitamin C can to a small degree significantly lower blood pressure. Vitamin C is also involved in the healthy function of mucous membranes, hormone production, phagocytosis and immune function. These are all activities which are of benefit when fighting cancer.

There have been laboratory studies using cancer cell lines in vitro where increased vitamin C levels caused a decrease in cell division and growth in a dosage-linked manner. These decreases occurred through the linked increase in the production of hydrogen peroxide.

Some studies have shown a protective association between vitamin C intake and the risk of prostate cancer. Notably advocates of increased Vitamin C intake included Linus Pauling a world famous quantum chemist and molecular biologist who won not just one but two Nobel Prizes and died aged 93 of prostate cancer which he believed he had managed for many years using vitamin C intravenously.

Vitamin D

One of the forgotten effects of reduced daylight hours during the winter months is the impact on vitamin D levels following reduced exposure to sunlight, and the negative result this can have on our health. Professor Michael Besser, London Consultant Endocrinologist "Vitamin D is of the utmost importance to your body, but deficiency is a very common – and little appreciated - problem in the UK. Current evidence suggests that about half of the population has insufficient levels, and the long-term impact to health is potentially debilitating. Whilst this is a particular issue during the winter, vitamin D deficiency is in fact a year-round epidemic that needs addressing."

Vitamin D is important for general good health, growth, strong bones, muscle function and immune response. The role of vitamin D is to assist your body to use the calcium and phosphorus obtained from your food. It also regulates normal cellular differentiation, thus helping to prevent cancer.

The great majority of our vitamin D is made in the skin with the help of sunlight, where UVB rays convert cholesterol into vitamin D, with the remaining amount obtained via a healthy diet. Exposure to sunlight can be reduced under cloud cover, and also in the shade, and the UVB rays are completely blocked by glass. Whilst challenges to gaining direct exposure are especially significant during the dark and dreary winter months, there are also challenges throughout the summer period with the increased use of sunblock. If exposure to the sun is limited, deficiency can occur, and this can eventually lead to osteomalacia – a disease that causes the bones to become weak and painful. Other associated conditions include muscle weakness, an increased risk of diabetes, heart disease and certain cancers.

Many different groups are more at risk of Vitamin D deficiency than others, in particular pregnant women, babies and people with black or Asian skin types.

Vitamin D is made by the body following exposure of the skin to sunlight. There is less sunlight in the UK than in southerly Mediterranean countries and also due to the temperature less opportunity to expose a large amount of your skin to sunlight.

It is one factor that may explain the higher levels of cancer in Northern Europeans than in Mediterranean Europeans. It is another important factor in combination with diet that would help explain the difference in cancer prevalence.

There is a danger linked to too much vitamin D of hypercalcaemia (too much calcium). Equally if getting Vitamin D through exposure to sunlight precautions are necessary to avoid the harmful effects of sunlight. This precaution is obviously extremely important if your cancer is a melanoma for example.

Vitamin D occurs naturally in animal foods as the pre- or pro-vitamin, cholecalciferol. This requires conversion in the kidney, which converts cholecalciferol to the active form of vitamin D known as Calcitriol. It is widely accepted that Calcitriol is very effective in reducing the proliferation of cancer cells. Alongside this ability to slow cancer growth there is increasing research evidence that vitamin D can play an important role in cancer treatment and prevention.

It has also been seen that Vitamin D helps to reduce the invasion of healthy cells by cancer cells as well as reduce the chances of metastases. Vitamin D seems to have a wide multifunction role in cancer treatment as it also appears to interfere with cancer cells at a molecular level by making their adhesion molecules less effective. Vitamin D also manages to enhance natural cell death (apoptosis) of cancer cells in a range of ways. If this wasn't enough Vitamin D also interferes with cancer cells ability to develop a blood supply (angiogenesis), which is very important as it means that the cancer cells will be less able to grow and divide.

Vitamin E

Vitamin E is in fact a group of fat-soluble phenols. Vitamin E supplements appear to reduce the risk of heart disease which as previously mentioned is considered an inflammatory disease. There are many different types of vitamin E. The one considered the most important in terms of oxidative stress management in humans is the fat-soluble antioxidant Alpha-Tocopherol. Wheat germ and sunflower oil have high levels. It is very useful in the management of ROS which are formed during lipid peroxidation. Alpha-Tocopherol is an important antioxidant which is heavily involved in the enzyme action of glutathione peroxidase. This action means that it is directly involved in the protection of cell membranes from ROS.

Many physiological functions, including those of the immune system are affected by the aging process. Normal immune functions are critical for healthy living in a modern world full of toxic chemicals and foreign organisms, but also good immune function is essential for protection from internally made toxic chemicals, cancers (cells acting as a foreign organism) and autoimmune diseases. Uncontrolled immune and inflammatory responses have been noted as more common in aging humans. This makes older people more susceptible and vulnerable to infectious diseases. Uncontrolled Inflammation has been considered to be one of the possible linked causes to many illnesses related to aging such as heart disease, rheumatoid arthritis, osteoporosis diabetes, Alzheimer's disease and Parkinson's disease. Therefore deeper research of oxidative stress and managing uncontrolled inflammation could hold the key to improved health in old age and cancer control

Vitamin E has many physiological functions within the body but its antioxidant function is the most important to consider during your fight against cancer. Vitamin E's link with inflammatory diseases and repair has been noted by many researchers and also Vitamin E supplements can help to lower blood cholesterol levels. Vitamin E is also known to be influential in connective tissue repair by its interaction with the connective tissue growth factor gene. When activated this gene is important in the repair of wounds and damage caused by atherosclerosis.

Vitamin E naturally occurs in eight different forms as the tocopherols (alpha, beta, gamma, and delta) and tocotrienols (alpha, beta, gamma, and delta), all of which possess powerful antioxidant properties. Gamma-tocopherol is the main type of vitamin E in the human diet, yet most studies have focused on the alpha-tocopherol type, which is the type found in most over-the-counter supplements.

Lab cell studies have shown decreased proliferation and increased apoptotic activity of vitamin E on prostate cancer cells. There are different prostate cancer cell types which react to the male hormone, androgen, differently but all gave increased apoptosis with alpha-tocopherol and vitamin E.

In living animal studies, vitamin E has been shown to inhibit prostate cancer growth in rats and mice. In the Alpha-Tocopherol, Beta-Carotene Cancer Prevention Study there was a 32% drop in the incidence of prostate cancer among people receiving alpha-tocopherol and a 41% drop in mortality from prostate cancer. This study also showed however that excessive, alpha-tocopherol was linked to an increased risk of bleeding in men with high blood pressure. In other studies men, who smoked but also took large amounts of vitamin E supplements had a greater than 40% drop in risk of advanced prostate cancer.

Selenium

Selenium is a mineral that is absorbed from the diet via plants. Its level in food depends on the selenium content of soil and water where the plants are grown. Selenium is found in the body as selenomethionine or selenocysteine in proteins. It is essential for glutathione peroxidase activity. Glutathione peroxidase is a useful enzyme that helps protect cells from oxidative damage and therefore reduces high levels of oxidative damage.

Test-tube studies have shown tumour growth inhibition with selenium. It seems clinical studies show that selenium has more of a protective ability than a pure treatment effect whilst slowing progression in some cancers. In the double-blind trial of dietary selenium supplementation carried out in the Nutritional Prevention of Cancer Study, a, selenium treatment was associated with a significant (63%) reduction in the secondary end point of prostate cancer incidence.

A detailed and longitudinal study of 9,345 Japanese-American men reviewed over 20 years showed men who had higher levels of selenium in their blood had a 50% drop in their risk of prostate cancer.

Jobs to do

1. Consider your vitamin and mineral intake and discuss with your dietician and oncologist especially Vitamin C and Selenium.

Chapter 5: Almonds

Almonds have been eaten by Mediterranean people for many, many years. In fact it has been held in high regard by humans throughout the ages, so much so that is mentioned in the Bible, Genesis 43:11 as "...among the best of fruits" and because of their supposed purity and protective qualities they are featured in paintings circling the baby Jesus. It is considered so highly that in Kashmir it is designated as the state tree. Evidence of cultivated almonds has been found in archaeological sites as early as the Bronze Age. Almonds were thought to be so important that they were buried along with other riches with the Pharaoh Tutankhamun (c. 1325 BC).

The trees are in fact native to the Middle East bordering the Mediterranean Sea. Almonds are very nutritious containing protein, carbohydrates, riboflavin, dietary fibre and key minerals such as manganese, magnesium copper, phosphorus, and calcium. In addition they have a high content of vitamin E and the monounsaturated fats, which is good at helping to lower Low Density Lipid (LDL) cholesterol levels.

One particular part of their protein make-up is the essential amino acid called tryptophan. It is called an essential amino acid as it is required by the human body but cannot be made (synthesized) by it and so must be eaten. It is also an essential amino acid because it has many uses including in the production of Serotonin, a highly important neurotransmitter in its own right but also an important signaling chemical for other key chemicals. Increased levels of tryptophan and the associated increase in serotonin is thought to aid a sense of well-being but also to aid restful sleep which are both very important in the fight against cancer. Anti-depressant drugs known as Selective Serotonin Re-uptake Inhibitors (SSRIs) increase the availability of serotonin. It is very interesting recent scientific studies have shown that increases in available serotonin levels are linked with significant impacts on the immune system and the inflammatory process. In particular these studies have shown a controlling impact on such key chemicals in many cancer processes as of Interferon-gamma (IFN-gamma), InterLeukin-6 (IL-6), InterLeukin-10 (IL-10) and Tumour Necrosis Factor (TNF). These studies lend support to the belief by many complimentary therapies that state of mind can play an important part in the outcomes of cancer sufferers. Clearly there is a great deal more study required before recommending wide-spread use of SSRIs in cancer therapy but this can be useful information for guiding your cancer fighting diet regime. Tryptophan is also used by the body in the production of Melatonin and Niacin commonly known as vitamin B3 both of which are also of key importance in the fight against cancer (see chapter on oxidative stress and B vitamins for more details).

Several recent research studies have found that by substituting animal fat in the subject's diet with almonds or almond oil, that significant reductions in total cholesterol levels and low-density lipoproteins (LDLs) were achieved. This occurs whilst the levels of high-density lipoproteins (HDLs) stayed relatively constant, which is good news. It has been seen following dietary studies involving almonds that there is a reduction in oxidative damage to proteins. Regular eating of almonds does not lead to an increase in weight, in fact eating them as part of a low-calorie diet promotes more weight loss than other similar low-calorie diets. Almonds seem to help humans in more ways than their immediate biochemical make-up would indicate as studies looking at obesity have found that increased intake of almonds has led to a reduced retention of nutrients and thus aiding complex weight loss programmes. The vitamin E levels within the blood is increased with increased almond intake, which with its antioxidant properties should help reduce oxidative damage at a wide range of sites and be especially helpful to the liver during its detoxification work.

The Food and Drug Administration (FDA) of the U.S.A. is widely known as being highly conservative in making health claims in general, but in 2003 felt that the body of evidence was sufficiently robust and overwhelming that it has allowed packages of almonds to carry health claims stating that scientific evidence suggests that eating 1.5 ounces per day of most nuts, such as almonds, as part of a diet low in saturated fat and cholesterol may reduce the risk of heart disease.

Following sustained interest in almonds and an effort to understand their impact on inflammatory processes researchers have identified the key chemicals that are responsible. This was done using state of the art techniques including High Performance Liquid Chromatography and tandem mass spectrometry. The other key ingredients are a mixture flavonoids and phenolic acids.

According to the U.S. Department of Agriculture nutrient database, whole almonds can yield weight for weight the highest natural levels of isorhamnetin, kaempferol, catechin, quercetin and epicatechin. These flavonoids may explain almonds significant health benefits especially in managing oxidative damage generally, but in the fight against cancer in particular the oxidative damage to DNA. Almond skins contain at least 30 different antioxidant compounds, including catechin, epicatechin, isorhamnetin, quercetin, and kaempferol. Quercetin especially has shown interesting antioxidant and antimutagenic properties.

There is increasing interest in the impact eating almonds have immediately after and research indicates that almonds might play a part in helping to manage diabetes and heart disease. There is reduced blood glucose noted quickly after eating almonds which could be helpful in reducing the risk of hypertension, diabetes and heart disease in people with a high risk. One theory of how this reduction in blood glucose occurs is that they lower the production of reactive oxygen species (ROS). In the absence of sufficient antioxidants, ROS may denature lipids, proteins and DNA. Analysis of almonds shows they contain high levels of antioxidants, also almonds due to their fat and protein levels could reduce blood glucose levels and therefore ROS production.

Increased blood glucose levels means that more is available for mitochondria to use and a linked increase in oxidative damage to proteins by ROS. The link to the important chemical sulphur is that ROS damage proteins by oxidizing their sulphur groups. Disulphide bonds are made in sulphur containing molecules like cysteine, methionine and glutathione. A drop in protein thiol concentrations can therefore be used as a marker of oxidative stress. Studies have shown that thiols are decreased in pathologies associated with increased oxidative stress, such as diabetes and autoimmune diseases. Thiol levels are notably reduced in cases of active systemic lupus erythematosus and were increased in diabetes after antioxidant supplementation. Recent studies indicate that the effect of antioxidants given as supplements in an attempt to reduce heart disease has largely been unsuccessful and so clearly as always the most common pathologies appear to be multi-factorial.

To gain the full benefit of almonds it is best to eat them raw (obviously without their shells) with their skins. Clearly on top of a handful of almonds a day you could indulge in a pasanda-style curry which includes cooked almonds. The additional benefit of a curry containing turmeric and aiding digestive transit should help also minimize oxidative damage within the colon. It is important that you do not eat almonds if you are allergic to nuts as although it is officially a fruit seed like that in a plum or peach it has nut-like allergies for some people. The usual advice applies that you should consult your doctor if unsure. This being said many people allergic to nuts can happily tolerate almonds in a range of forms. The health benefits in the fight against cancer are like many areas still needing more extensive research but there are small human and animal studies yielding encouraging results also in other inflammatory diseases such as diabetes and heart disease.

Jobs to do

1. Go to shop today and buy enough almonds for a handful a day for the next month and put around your house in small bowls to remind you to eat them. By the kettle and TV remote are good starting places so is next to your computer and in your car.

2. Celebrate by going out for a take-away a passanda curry or buying a ready-made one from the shops. If you are a great cook then if you like make your own but this is hardly a celebration of your new love for almonds.

Chapter 6: The Tomato or Golden Apple

The tomato's health benefits have resurfaced in recent years but in fact its properties were well known and even written about in Europe in the 16th century. The Italian doctor and botanist, Pietro Mattioli, is credited with first researching and publishing its health benefits. He was so impressed by it that he called it "pomo d'oro", which is still the Italian word used for tomato. Pomo d'oro translates literally as golden apple and it appears that it may have rightly been given such a name in terms of its value to the Italian diet, but also its valuable health benefits.

The links between health benefits for cancer sufferers and cardiovascular disease and the Mediterranean diet seems to continue with the tomato. There has been a lot of research activity regarding the health benefits of tomatoes especially processed tomatoes which is not only biochemical but also clinical in nature. The health benefits of tomatoes are believed to be linked to a carotenoid present in tomatoes called lycopene. However there is a very wide range of tomato varieties and it is important to remember that they also contain other antioxidants such as anthocyanin and carotene in differing amounts. Remembering that all vegetables and fruit are good generally, if not poisonous and free from disease, additives etc., it seems rather simplistically that the more colourful ones are more beneficial. Carotenoids like lycopene are important pigments found in photosynthetic pigment-protein complexes in plants, photosynthetic bacteria, fungi, and algae. They are responsible for the bright colors of fruits and vegetables, perform various functions in photosynthesis, and protect photosynthetic organisms from excessive light damage. Lycopene is a key intermediate in the biosynthesis of many important carotenoids, such as beta-carotene.

Like other carotenoids, lycopene is a natural pigment synthesized by plants and microorganisms but not by animals. It is not however made by humans and so must be eaten. It occurs in the human diet predominantly in tomatoes and processed tomato products. It is yet another antioxidant but is a very powerful one and is in fact the best of all carotenoids at protecting cells from the damage caused by "free-radicals."

Carotenoid pigments are essential in the fight against cancer and especially the damage caused by free radicals and in particular singlet oxygen. In plants during photosynthesis, it is common for singlet oxygen to be produced by chlorophyll molecules. One of the roles of carotenoids in plants is to prevent the damage caused by singlet oxygen. Carotenoids do this by either limiting excess UV light energy from chlorophyll molecules or by neutralizing the singlet oxygen molecules directly.

This connection between cancer and cardiovascular problems appears to be linked to the damage of singlet oxygen causes which is produced during the oxidation of Low Density Lipoprotein-Cholesterol (LDL-C). LDL-C is often referred to as the bad cholesterol due to its links to cardiovascular problems. Therefore anything such as lycopene that can neutralize these highly reactive oxygen species is considered beneficial, hence the significant interest in antioxidants which can reduce the levels of these dangerous substances.

Given its antioxidant properties, substantial scientific and clinical research has been devoted to a possible link between lycopene consumption and general health. Research indicates that lycopene can have a positive impact on a range of conditions but especially on heart disease, diabetes and cancer.

The effects of lycopene on prostate cancer have been studied by many different researchers both clinically-based and laboratory-based researchers found that lycopene has a significant impact and a protective benefit. These studies have been of substantial size and controlled and are widely accepted within the research community. These tomato-based health benefits continued even after accounting for other fruit and vegetable consumption. Among the standard tomato-based products considered, the link was strongest for tomato sauce.

Lycopene is a non-provitamin A carotenoid and is the most efficient singlet-oxygen (a Reactive Oxygen Species = ROS) quencher among the natural carotenoids. ROS will be covered in much more detail in the oxidative stress chapters which follow. Lycopene may be considered to be one of the most powerful neutralizers of free radicals (singlet oxygen molecules) brought about due to oxidative stress. It appears in some lab tests to be 10,000 % more capable than Vitamin E and even more again than glutathione.

Lycopene when chemically isolated is a bright red colour and gives many plants' fruits and vegetables their red colour. Lycopene is a predominantly plant pigment. It is found in very high levels in a fruit called gac and high levels in tomatoes but also to a much lesser degree in many other red fruits and vegetables. Gac is the king of lycopene content with approximately at least twenty times the content weight for weight over tomato juice. Following tests by the US Department of Agriculture (USDA) they confirmed in the *Journal of Agricultural and Food Chemistry* (2004, Vol. 52, pp 274-279), extracts from the gac fruit also contain 40 times the zeaxanthin in corn, and is a source of omega-6 and omega-9 fatty acids, and vitamin E. This is great but it has only had limited availability around the world, rarely used outside of Vietnam and until recently is highly priced. This may change when its full benefits are realised and understood. There is little direct scientific research of its actual capabilities and so tomato wins the lycopene-containing fruit of choice on grounds of the amount of research done and the evidence-base of health benefits. However if you feel the need to try it is available on the internet as a dietary supplement. Clearly if lycopene is the sole key ingredient in tomatoes cancer-fighting properties and high levels result in health benefits then it might be worth a try but this is a leap of faith not based on substantial direct research of the gac fruit and its extracts. I personally am happy to reserve judgement as lots of things that are highly researched still turn out to be far from perfect for certain uses (such as thalidomide) and equally the converse is true. It is likely that Gac due to its very high lycopene content as well as other reported health benefits may become more widely researched and therefore more widely used in time. If your fight against cancer is particularly difficult and you seem to be definitely losing it is definitely worth a try even though there is limited research.

There have been several studies produced that analyze the anti-cancer properties of lycopene. Evidence for lycopene's benefit was strongest for cancers of the lung, stomach, and prostate gland. Lycopene is not converted to vitamin A in the body unlike other pre-cursors. This means that the body can use lycopene to its fullest degree in the battle against cancer and free radicals. Lycopene is the main carotenoid throughout the body on the whole. Lycopene has also been found present in the lungs with cancer where it is used by the body to protect the lymphocytes thus supporting the immune and inflammatory response. Although some people who are not used to consuming higher levels of processed tomatoes may find increased and watery bowel movements it is also possible that lycopene helps lower the damage caused by free radicals from infections in the stomach. There is a fair degree of support for the belief that lycopene may help reduce the risk and growth of cancer by activating special cancer preventive enzymes such as phase II detoxification enzymes, which remove toxins from cells and the body. It has been seen that it arrests growth of certain cancers such as endometrial cancer. This linked with its ability to block an insulin-like growth factor which is a key component of the control of cell growth especially in breast, womb, colon and prostrate tissue tends to indicate that it really is big player on the list of dietary components that can really help in the fight against cancer.

Lycopene is found and transported in blood by various lipoproteins throughout the body however it is often found in larger concentrations in fatty tissues and organs e.g. the kidneys, adrenal glands, liver, breast, testes etc.). After ingestion, lycopene becomes incorporated into lipid formations within the gut which helps the lycopene to become absorbed through the gut wall and into the lymphatic system also, where it is believed they make a significant impact.

Although lycopene is chemically a carotene, it is not a pre-cursor for Vitamin A like other carotenoids. This is important to understand as high intakes of Vitamin A in the form of supplements has been associated by some with higher risk of lung cancer in smokers and those exposed to other airborne toxic substances such as asbestos. Lycopene is considered non-toxic and so its red colour is put to use in processed foods as a natural E-number colouring. As previously mentioned lycopene is edible and considered non-toxic. Even high level intakes appear to have limited long term negative effects reported. However if lycopene is taken to excess in humans the pigment is so strong that in fact the skin can discolour. Lycopene is not a required foodstuff for humans to live healthily, but as already stated is very helpful and mainly comes from food prepared with processed tomatoes in it.

Cooking and crushing tomatoes such as in canning and serving in oil-rich dishes (such as pasta or pizza sauces greatly increases assimilation from the digestive tract into the bloodstream. Lycopene is fat-soluble, so the oil helps absorption into the body from the gut. Major population studies have shown that when compare to other antioxidants, only high lycopene intake or plasma concentrations are associated with a lower risk of prostate cancer. For example, consumption of four or five servings of tomato products per week was associated with a 40% lower risk of prostate cancer in men. The exact way which lycopene reduces prostate cancer risk is still not fully agreed. However Lycopene has been shown to reduce extreme cell division in various cancer cell lines.

Many studies including placebo-controlled studies using a randomized, cross-over design of tomato-based products eaten by humans have looked at the antioxidant properties of lycopene. They have found that blood serum and prostrate levels of lycopene were significantly higher following increased intake of tomato-based products or lycopene supplements. They also found that cellular proteins and lymphocytes' (important White Blood Cells - WBCs) DNA were less damaged due to oxidative damage. It is noted that lycopene concentrations in human lymphocytes increased by almost 50% following a short period of increased consumption and along with that there was approximately a 50% reduction DNA strand breaks (DNA damage) in the lymphocytes following exposure to oxidants. It is likely that with increased concentrations of lycopene in different tissue (e.g. prostrate, breast, liver etc.) that a similar reduction in DNA damage may be possible.

Free radicals and ROS in general are believed to play a critical role in all stages of carcinogenesis due to oxidative damage to DNA. This DNA damage can lead to faster cell growth and poorer use or availability of DNA repair enzymes. Oxidative damage to the DNA chemical 2_-deoxyguanosine (dG) by singlet oxygen turns it into 8-hydroxy- 2-deoxyguanosine (8-OHdG). 8-OHdG is therefore the most prevalent DNA damage chemical and when it becomes part of the DNA complex it leads to mutation and therefore possibly cancer. Increased 8-OHdG levels have been noted in several different cancer tissues and in human leucocytes from people with different diseases linked with oxidative damage. Lower 8-OHdG levels have also been noted in human leukocytes from people eating foods high in antioxidants including tomatoes. Oxidative damage is noted by lower levels of a chemical called 8-hydroxy-2-deoxyguanosine or 8-OHdG for short in comparison to the levels of 2-deoxyguanosine (dG). ROS and in particular singlet oxygen is a major generator of 8-OhdG, which is why it is often monitored as a marker for oxidative damage. It has been found that this ratio 8-OhdG to dG chemical levels in circulating lymphocytes is possibly a good marker of oxidative damage caused by many cancers which impact on oxidative damage to the liver and has also in fact been seen to be high in people with liver diseases such as hepatitis. Interestingly there are also reduced levels of thiobarbituric acid-reactive chemicals in the blood serum following an increase in consumption of tomato-based products or lycopene supplements.

A large number of well-designed studies have shown that there is significant benefit in increased consumption of lycopene over a short period with lower leukocyte DNA damage a major part of that which can aid in the fight against cancer. Placebo and blinded studies on processed tomato products have been carried out which confirm many others positive findings. Results have shown 100% increase in lycopene serum concentration and it is estimated up to a 300% increase in lycopene prostrate tissue concentration.

If eaten regularly tomato products have been suspected to cause stomach ache for some people, so if you do not already eat a lot of tomato-based products it is a good idea to keep a watchful eye out for this if you start to try increasing your dietary intake of tomato-based products. A few people have reported an increase in stomach aches linked with increased incidence of gas, burping and heartburn following increasing their tomato products intake. For those people who suffer with stomach ache or do not wish to eat tomato-based products daily there are lycopene supplements which are an easy way to take lycopene regularly.

The evidence from studies overwhelmingly suggests that prostate cancer patients have high prostate DNA damage that may be reduced with tomato sauce consumption. Tomato paste and sauces seem to yield the best results of biologically available lycopene. Even though tomato paste and sauces contains many antioxidants, it is accepted that lycopene is the most active compound because of its impact on ROS.

There is significant evidence that tomato-based products, containing lycopene, reduce the compounds present due to oxidative stress a believed cause of prostrate hyperplasia and cancer growth in patients especially those with prostate cancer. It has also been considered beneficial in people with lung, stomach, breast and head and neck cancers. There has also been evidence to show health benefits for certain types of diabetes. Although we tend to think in health and diet terms that "fresh is best", it appears that this is far from the case when regarding the health benefits of tomatoes. Studies have shown that processed tomato products like tomato juice, tomato paste, tomato puree and even tomato ketchup provide better levels of absorbable lycopene than the same amount of fresh produce. Lycopene is insoluble in water and is in fact highly integrated into tomato fibre and so it is believed that these different forms of processing help to make it more absorbable by the body. In fact processed tomato products such as tomato juice, soup, sauce, and ketchup contain the highest concentrations of lycopene from tomato products. It has also been found that normally available edible fats help the body even more with the absorption of lycopene and so edible fats should be eaten at the same time. These edible fats could be in the form of olive oil which links again nicely with the anti-cancer benefits of the Mediterranean diet again.

It appears that lycopene from tomatoes help protect proteins from damage due to excess free radicals arising from oxidative stress. The protected proteins which are key to human physiological performance include lipoproteins and white blood cell (lymphocyte) DNA. It also appears that lycopene from tomatoes have anticarcinogenic properties which cause reduction in antigens and tumour growth especially prostate tumours.

Lycopene has such strong pigment properties and ultra-violet light protection properties that reasonable levels within the body has also been shown to improve the skin's ability to protect against harmful UV rays and thus potentially aid the body's protection from skin cancers.

Obviously just because you are eating tomatoes does not mean you can sunbathe without adequate protection in the form of sun creams, hats etc. especially if you are white skinned, blue/green eyed and blonde or red-haired. The other good news surrounding regular tomato consumption is it leads to increased levels of pro-collagen, a protein which helps give skin its tone and youthfulness. Therefore not only are you improving your cancer protection and fighting chances and further protecting your skin from sun damage but also you may even stop your skin from looking so old as it would do. Fighting cancer and looking pretty! Who would have thought all this would be possible from the humble tomato maybe if we named it the golden apple it would be given the respect it deserves.

It makes sense that eating processed tomato products, containing lycopene, is a significant help in fighting cancer. This links in with the Mediterranean diet theory of reduced cancer risk, which has tomatoes as a common element of the Mediterranean diet. So if you like food with lots of processed tomatoes, such as Spanish or Italian for example then you are in luck and if you like tomato ketchup then this component of your fight against cancer is easy. Remember that lycopene is not water soluble and so make sure that you have it with oil. I personally think due to its high levels of polyphenols, link to the Mediterranean diet and taste that olive oil is the best.

Have a tomato juice to start the day, every day with a half shot glass of olive oil. If that gets a bit boring, why not try a Bloody Mary by including a small nip of vodka, a few drops of Tabasco, a glug of Worcester sauce and a stick of celery. With that inside you every morning you are sure to be happier every morning but clearly be careful if expecting to drive or use machinery later. Also please be conscious of the impact of alcohol on any other medication you may be taking. Even as little as five tablespoons of tomato paste added to the diet with naturally occurring fats or oils can have a significant effect in 60 days if taken daily. This could be used in cooking ideally or taken directly from the tube or jar. You could make your own pizzas, Bolognese etc. or just add extra tomato paste and olive oil to shop bought pre-made ready to cook purchases for ease. It is important to have some naturally occurring fats too as lycopene is fat-soluble and so this aids the effective absorption of the lycopene into the body.

Jobs to do

1. Go to the shops and buy lots of tomato ketchup, sauces, purees and pastes and aim to use daily in your cooking and eating if possible. Processed tomato sauces appear to give high levels of lycopene but why not add all together and make your own sauce of sauces. Who knows if it is really good you could market it and compete with Dolmio! If not then squeeze a large mouthful of tomato paste in your mouth from a tube or have a small portion of steamed vegetables or oven chips with lots of tomato ketchup or a bowl of pasta/spaghetti with passata or tinned tomatoes and olive oil.

2. Clearly you could buy lycopene supplements instead which you could take daily after discussion with your oncologist.

Chapter 7: What is Oxidative Stress? - A key area of scientific interest in the fight against cancer.

I am not sure I can explain it simply but I will give it my best shot. As always there is loads of info on the internet with some very good stuff but not always put simply. Usually as soon as we mention the words Chemistry, Biology and Physics many of us think back to our school days of boring lessons which had little relevance to our day-to-day lives, however I think it is highly useful to have a grasp of these if we are to understand how best to help ourselves fight cancer using modern science and complimentary medicine including dietary supplements.

We will start with a review of the fundamentals as it should help us understand some of the terms and ideas which follow. I have tried to give you a fair amount of detail whilst keeping it interesting. If you find yourself getting bored or getting a headache whilst reading you have my permission to skip this chapter and head straight to the end to the "**Jobs to Do**" section. Don't worry too much if you find this section too difficult to understand as with all science most times you do not have to understand it completely to benefit from it. Just like you do not need to know how a petrol engine works to use a car, you do not need to fully understand how smoking causes cancer to gain the health benefits from not smoking. Strangely apart from the tar and other toxins it is believed that the high levels of oxidants in cigarette smoke are one of the main causes of cancers related to smoking, because of the increased oxidative stress lung cells etc. are put under. Anyway to get back to the point all you need to do in life with almost everything is to make a considered decision on the information available to you.

Clearly I will try to keep it brief and to the point without skipping too many important points. I hope to make it interesting for you with a fair amount of detail, but for those of you who find this whole area intriguing there is plenty of detail in other books and on the web to digest but in particular I would like to recommend the very detailed review published in the Toxicologic Pathology journal by Ron Kohen and Abraham Nyska (see references).

Oxidation & Reduction Explained
So to start with if we forget about discussions relating to our souls and theology for a minute, then we humans are but a chemical bag of chemicals. Clearly humans in my humble opinion, on the whole, are of course very beautiful and finely balanced bags of chemicals, but chemical bags of chemicals none the less. The human body is composed of cells and for our bodies to work efficiently its cells need oxygen and food to convert to usable energy. Oxygen as we know is essential for our survival, but there is a lot of stuff we don't know or remember about oxygen.

The discovery of oxygen is usually credited to Joseph Priestly in 1774 due to his publication of a paper however others such as Antoine Laurent Lavoisier and Carl Wilhelm Scheele were highly instrumental in our understanding of oxygen with Carl Wilhelm Scheele, a Swedish chemist probably being the actual first person to discover oxygen. In fact the name oxygen was given by Lavoisier and comes from Greek and means acid producer. This is a good reminder of one of its potentially toxic properties because although oxygen is an essential requirement for human life it can also be detrimental. In fact Priestley also described the toxic effects of pure oxygen in 1775. It took many years for a fuller understanding of oxygen to emerge. To put this in perspective it was found that too much oxygen in the 1940s was being given to premature babies in their newly invented incubators. This led to toxic effects of too much oxygen becoming apparent with blindness being one of the worst.

I will attempt to explain oxidation and reduction in some detail but hopefully in a way that makes sense and also shows its importance in helping to win the fight against cancer both in terms of prevention and treatment.

In simple terms oxidation is simply chemical reactions where oxygen is involved. Like many chemical reactions there are byproducts or waste products also released during oxidation. These like most waste products can be toxic especially with increased concentration. The term oxidation became more complicated in so far as the meaning of oxidation expanded to involve chemical reactions which involved the "loss" of at least one electron when two or more chemicals react. These chemicals may or may not include oxygen. The opposite of oxidation is reduction, which is a reaction involving the loss of oxygen. Just for balance reduction is also considered the addition of at least one electron when chemicals react with each other. These electrons do not just end up flying around by themselves for long periods of time but find a new home very quickly which is usually a new molecule or new atom. Therefore the two reactions occur together to all intense purposes with some chemical losing an electron (oxidation) and another chemical gaining an electron (reduction). This is why you may hear people refer to redox reactions which is short for reduction and oxidation reactions. Generally reductant and oxidant are terms used to describe the chemicals in Chemistry, but in Biochemistry they are more often referred to as antioxidant and pro-oxidant. Pro-oxidants that have oxygen as a key reactive component are called reactive oxygen species (ROS). I will refer to ROS predominantly throughout and it will be implied that they are the more significant free radicals unless clarified due to the damaging power of the ROS free radicals superoxide, hydroxyl radical and hydrogen peroxide. Free radicals are any short-lived and highly reactive chemical whether in an atomic, molecular or ionic form. Free radicals are atoms or groups of atoms with an uneven number of electrons and can be formed when oxygen interacts with certain molecules. Once formed these highly reactive radicals can start a chain reaction. They can damage human cells when they react with important cellular components such as DNA or the cell membrane. All cellular membranes are especially vulnerable to oxidation damage due to their high concentrations of unsaturated fatty acid. The damage to lipids is via the reaction called lipid peroxidation. Proteins are also major constituents of membranes and can also be possible targets for attack by ROS. Some of the possible consequences of protein damage can be loss of enzymatic activity, altered cellular functions such as energy production, interference with the creation of membrane potentials, and changes in the types of proteins. Protein oxidation products can also be dangerous to the cell such as aldehydes and carbonyls.

Cells can often not function so well or even die if this occurs. To limit free radical damage to cells, the body has a defence system of antioxidants. For most cells free radical damage is closely related to oxidation/oxidative damage. In human biology the key free radicals are often referred to as Reactive Oxygen Species (ROS) because the most biologically important free radicals have a key oxygen component. However not all free radicals are ROS and not all ROS are free radicals. Free radicals play an important part in many essential cellular processes. These processes include the killing of bacteria by White Blood Cells and "cell signaling" such as signaling natural cell growth or death. It is accepted that large concentrations of free radicals can lead to unnatural cell growth, cell injury or even cell death. These detrimental cell effects can lead to a range of diseases including serious inflammatory conditions such as diabetes, arthritis, heart disease, strokes and cancer. Reactions between DNA and free radicals occur and it is widely accepted that this can lead to mutations which in turn can lead to cancer formation. It is also believed that free radicals are directly involved in alcohol-related liver damage, Parkinson's and Alzheimer's diseases as well as many others. The human body needs the actions of free radicals for normal life but due to their highly reactive and potentially damaging effects it has a complex system to manage them and repair any damage free radicals cause. This system involves the use enzymes such as **superoxide dismutase, catalase, glutathione peroxidase and reductase and also the use of antioxidants such as Vitamins A, C & E and polyphenol antioxidants.** Oxidative stress and subsequent damage occur when this management system cannot cope with the concentration, location and/or type of free radicals.

In the 1950s a free radical theory of cellular aging was proposed by Denham Harman, which has been supported by many researchers and updated to move away slightly from the aging theory but to focus on the damage that free radicals can do to cell structures and their relationship to diseases. Simply it is the gentle natural balance between acceptable oxidative stress and unacceptable oxidative damage which is the body's main job to avoid cancer. Many researchers and clinicians accept that when there is significant imbalance leading to excessive oxidative stress that this can cause damage and mutation of the DNA to occur which can lead to cancer.

It appears that ROS produced during normal cell activity (cellular respiration) can cause cumulative damage which can eventually lead to loss of function. This link seems to continue with many traditionally age-related diseases such as arthritis, heart disease, diabetes and cancer. ROS and free radicals in general are key chemicals involved in normal cell death either programmed or not such as White Blood Cells (WBCs) ability to eat other foreign bodies, bacteria etc. and thereby maintain our immune system cells whilst also being involved in inflammation.

As we said earlier free radicals and especially ROS are highly reactive and so as a consequence can be indiscriminate in the chemicals they react with such as DNA. Because most radicals are short-lived species, they react quickly. Most ROS are extremely reactive. To give you an idea of how quickly they can react some ROS actually only exist for millionths of a second before they react, when they are created in living cells. How long ROS survive varies and does also depend on other factors such as Ph (how acidic or alkali a solution is). However it is important to be aware that just because a chemical is highly reactive and does so quickly does not mean it is more dangerous or toxic to the cell. It does also depend on where it occurs and how sensitive that region is to damage. Unfortunately oxidation during cellular metabolism occurs in the mitochondria which are in close proximity to the cell's DNA. Although DNA is a very stable, well-protected molecule, ROS can interact with it and cause several types of damage. This damage can range from changes to DNA bases to single- and double-DNA breaks and damage to the DNA repair system.

Clearly I am not saying that oxidative stress is the sole cause of cancer but I feel it plays a significant role in cellular efficiency and damage. According to Mosby's Medical Dictionary on the web, oxidative stress can be described as any of various pathologic changes seen in living organisms in response to excessive levels of cytotoxic oxidants and free radicals in the environment. Food stuffs or food supplements containing antioxidants can help to provide both preventively and therapeutically to reduce the damaging effects of free radicals and/or oxidants on cellular constituents. To put that more simply there are ways to reduce the cellular damage caused by free radicals (highly reactive chemicals within the body) by taking foods or supplements containing antioxidants / other naturally occurring chemicals that can directly or indirectly help to "neutralise" these free radicals.

Where do all these potentially dangerous chemicals or oxidants come from?

The simple answer is that a significant number and concentration are made by our own bodies. This will be explained in some detail below. The next major provider of ROS is our food, hence the focus on our diets throughout this book. There are several ways in which the reactive oxygen species (ROS) are found in or on the human body. Most occur as by-products of normal and essential metabolic chemical reactions. ROS also come from a range of outside sources from "pollutants" such as cigarette smoke, car and factory emissions, industries, certain herbicides and pesticides, excessive alcohol consumption, excessive narcotic consumption, asbestos, exposure to ionizing and non-ionising radiation (e.g. sunlight, x-rays and ultrasound), anaesthetic gases and bacterial, fungal or viral infections. For bacteria, fungi and viruses the increase in ROS can be as a natural by-product of their own metabolism or as a consequence of our own body's immune system and its White Blood Cells activity.

A significant amount of our food consumed is oxidised and contains many oxidants such as oxidised fatty acids, peroxides and transition metals. This could be why the gut and specifically the colon is so prone to cancer due to this often high level of oxidative stress which is also cumulative like cell metabolism.

Lots of diseases themselves are not only initiated by oxidative stress but also by their very nature increase production of ROS and thus increase oxidative stress. ROS seem to be highly important pre-cursors or signallers for many cancers as well as diabetes, inflammation, heart disease, degenerative brain diseases and other key organ degeneration such as liver and kidneys. The link to the aging process is due to an apparent increase in ROS production due to less effective mitochondrial function with age.

Antioxidants are highly influential in dealing with oxidants and therefore reducing oxidative stress. Antioxidants are a wide range of chemicals that protect cells against the damaging effects of Reactive Oxygen Species (ROS), such as superoxide, singlet oxygen, peroxyl radicals and hydroxyl radicals. We have talked already about antioxidant enzymes but we are now going to focus on edible antioxidants and their pre-cursors. The correct intake of antioxidants is highly desirable because a negative imbalance between antioxidants and reactive oxygen species results in oxidative stress, leading to cellular damage. Oxidative Stress and the associated damage that ROS causes, has meant that the use of antioxidants in cancer prevention and therapy has been researched fairly widely with many detailed studies. Obviously with all research areas there will be those for and those against recommending certain antioxidants. Antioxidants are believed to be effective in helping to prevent cancer, heart disease, stroke and a variety of other ailments associated with natural aging. There are many different types of cancers as well as many different types of antioxidants.

When our body cells use oxygen, they naturally produce ROS (by-products) which can cause damage. Antioxidants are often food-based chemicals that can stop or reduce oxidation and/or neutralize the effects of ROS. In humans, oxidative stress is linked directly and indirectly to a number of chronic diseases including cardiovascular disease and cancer. Antioxidants in foods are important to a healthy diet and steps can be taken to preserve the antioxidant content of foods. Keeping fruits and vegetables in a cool, dry place helps to slow down the natural breakdown by enzymes that begin to occur as soon as the foods are picked. There are many scientific advocates of the health benefits of fresh vegetable and fruit juices especially in the fight against cancer. Juicers have tripled in sales over that last two years based on the health benefits of fresh vegetable and fruit juices. Although the majority of these juices are packed with natural antioxidants people find it hard to get into the habit of buying and juicing fresh fruit and vegetables. The benefits cannot be understated and so one of your **Jobs to do** is to buy and use a juicer following many of the recipes available on the internet. Even though due to human nature just like bread-making machines these machines are often left unused after the first few weeks, it is still a worthwhile investment for your fight against cancer. Generally speaking people with cancer that want to fight it are a little more motivated than the general population and so if you use it daily as part of your sixty day routine then you have achieved a significant benefit.

Your own body has antioxidants and they exist naturally in many forms and help prevent oxidative damage to tissues. Oxidative damage is considered potentially significant in the development and growth of cancer, because of this, it has followed that antioxidants may help prevent cancer. Many studies suggest that people who eat more vegetables and fruits, which are rich sources of antioxidants (including vitamin C, vitamin E, carotenoids, and many other antioxidant phytochemicals), may have a lower risk for some types of cancer. It is essential that even if you are a cancer sufferer who has been successfully treated it is a good idea to have a selection of antioxidant-rich foods each day or take supplements as with many cancers you will be at increased risk of cancer returning.

Using antioxidants to reduce or heal diseases is far from accepted by all scientists and research studies. In fact one antioxidant appears to possibly have the reverse effect. When taken in significant amounts by smokers, beta-carotene was shown to increase the incidence of lung cancer in one study. To counteract oxidative stress, the body produces a significant range of antioxidants to defend itself from potential oxidative damage. Your body's ability to produce antioxidants is controlled to some degree by your genetic makeup and influenced by your exposure to environmental factors such as diet and smoking. The vitamins A, C, D & E are powerful antioxidants. There are many antioxidants which can be useful in the fight against cancer and probably a variety is more effective than excess of one particular one due to the body's ability to excrete excess and adapt to varying levels. Cancer cells are also body cells and it would appear that they are also able to adapt to their environment.

Like all things to do with the human body there are a large number of confounding variables which affect the impact that these oxidants and any subsequent oxidative stress will have on us as individuals which include how old we are, what our family and personal genetic history are, whether we are male or female, where we live, what we eat, what we do etc. etc.

First make a cup of tea which is ideally green tea and then relax and breathe in, as what follows may take some digesting mentally.

A human cell needs energy if it is to perform the required activities for living and for the full body to work well. We get the energy for our cells and us ultimately to live from food. This food is broken down and the energy within its chemical bonds is used. The energy within food's chemical bonds must be converted into something our bodies can readily use and so food's energy is used to help to convert adenosine diphosphate (ADP) into adenosine triphosphate (ATP). This is achieved using a chemical reaction pathway called oxidative phosphorylation. This set of chemical reactions is often referred to as the Citric Acid or the Krebs Cycle after the scientist that discovered it. This set of reactions occurs in the cell's mitochondria, which can be considered the power supply factories of the cell. A bit like a coal or oil-fuelled power plant mitochondria converts one form of energy into a more usable form of energy. The power plants have coal or oil with oxygen and convert their energy into electricity, whereas mitochondria have food (glucose) and oxygen and convert their energy into ATP. Unfortunately for us like most power stations the mitochondria are far from 100% clean and efficient and as part of their normal activity they create toxic waste in the form of highly reactive toxic chemicals. Again like most power stations cells have processes in place for managing this waste which a lot of the time work okay but are not perfect. This toxic waste management system can often become less reliable even leaky the older the power station and the greater the activity that is expected of it, just like mitochondria.

In simple terms ATP is another chemical form of energy that our bodies and cells can easily use. A quite interesting fact that is often quoted is that theoretically for every one glucose molecule that is oxidized by 6 oxygen molecules the energy released can help create 38 molecules of ATP. In reality as we and our cells are only human it is more often in reality around 30 molecules of ATP that are created, which is still pretty efficient. The ATP, which stores the energy, is used by the body to enable chemical processes requiring energy such as the manufacture of other chemicals (biosynthesis) or the active movement of chemicals across cell membranes or cell activity such as muscle cells contracting in the heart etc.

This ATP production process is often referred to as the metabolic breakdown of foodstuffs, our metabolism or sometimes cellular respiration or metabolism. It is often called cellular respiration because it occurs at a cellular level with the other chemical, which our cells need for life and this metabolism to occur, being oxygen. This type of metabolic breakdown of foodstuffs is also often referred to as aerobic respiration due to the involvement of oxygen. Our cells can perform anaerobic respiration which is the metabolic breakdown of foodstuffs without oxygen, but this method does not yield as much energy as with oxygen and also our cells cannot maintain this exclusively for very long periods due to the significant buildup of toxic waste products with this method. To give you an idea of how inefficient anaerobic respiration is using a chemical reaction pathway called glycolysis, only approximately 2 molecules of ATP are created per one glucose molecule, which is pretty inefficient when compared to the 30 possible when using oxygen in the oxidative phosphorylation method. The human body in areas of high energy consumption such as the brain and liver for example consumes large amounts of ATP as well as oxygen, which often leads to high levels of reactive oxygen species production as a by-product.

Oxidative Stress and Inflammation

One negative effect of oxidative stress is the beginning of a state of mild irregular inflammation. This type of mild inflammation is often present in many degenerative diseases linked with aging.

If you ever wonder why serious drug abusers look old and the way they do some of it appears to be due to oxidative stress. Usually serious drug abusers' diets are poor anyway but it now has been shown that cocaine and possibly other similar compounds help induce oxidative damage to the skin and lead to this premature aging effect.

Oxidative stress has been linked to heart disease and arthrosclerosis, as the oxidation of Low Density Lipoproteins (LDLs) occurs. Unfortunately LDLs help with the transport of cholesterol within blood vessels and oxidation of these LDLs can lead to cholesterol plaques "growing". This can lead to a very poor circulation. A good circulation of blood is essential in fighting any disease especially cancer and also ultimately these plaques lead to heart attacks and strokes.

Consistent oxidative stress with ROS production leads to the activation of a chemical, known as the "nuclear factor kappa-light-chain-enhancer of activated B cells" (NFkB). This is a seriously complex, complex protein and was found by David Baltimore, an American winner of the Nobel Prize in Physiology or Medicine. NFkB is a chemical complex that controls the movement (transcription) of genetic information within DNA and can cause pro-inflammatory activity. There is significant evidence that decreasing oxidative stress inhibits activation of NFkB.

Oxidative stress can and often does lead to activation of NFkB, which promotes transcription of pro-inflammatory genes that then have an impact on cell adhesion molecules such as intercellular adhesion molecule-1 (ICAM-1), enzymes such as nitric oxide synthase and cycloxygenase-2 (COX-2), cytokines, interleukin-6, interleukin-8 and chemokines. It has been noted by researchers that NFkB and COX-2 are active in Alzheimer's disease. NFkB activation is also seen in atherosclerosis, which is primarily an inflammatory disease. This inflammatory process is unfortunately progressive in nature. This inflammatory process leads to sticky molecules being created and deposited which in turn can lead to a less effective immune system due to white blood cells (leucocytes) sticking to blood vessels. This occurs especially where there are atherosclerotic plaques (fatty deposits) already present. Therefore if we consider this chain of events it should be possible to reduce the inflammatory process by limiting the activation of NFkB in the first place. This could be possible by improving the management of strong oxidants produced by cellular metabolism by the use of antioxidants.

NFkB is widely used by cells as a regulator of genes that control cell multiplication and cell survival. Many different types of human tumours have interfered with NFkB levels and production. High levels of activated NFkB turns on the expression of genes that keep the cell proliferating and protect the cell from conditions that would otherwise cause it to die via the normal process of cell death known as apoptosis. In cancer cells, NFkB is active due to mutations in genes responsible for NFkB activity. Even more "alien-like", some tumor cells secrete chemicals that cause NFkB to become active. It is widely accepted that by blocking NFkB activity we can cause tumor cells to stop, cause tumour cells to die and even to become more sensitive to traditional chemotherapy. Thus, NFkB is the subject of much active research among pharmaceutical companies as a target for anti-cancer therapy. NFkB interacts with lots of genes related to inflammation and so it is not unexpected that NFkB appears to be involved in many inflammatory diseases (e.g. inflammatory bowel disease, arthritis and asthma). It has been found that many chemicals from herbs and dietary plants are efficient inhibitors of NFkB.

The Vitamin Bs important links with Sulphur, Glutathione, Coenzyme A & NADH

You might think that we are going into too much detail but the Krebs Cycle and its efficiency can have significant health impacts. It is also important to realize that many chemicals involved in this series of reactions within the mitochondria need to be readily available to every cell in your body to maintain efficiency. Two of the most important chemicals are coenzyme A and NADH (Reduced form of Nicotinamide Adenine Dinucleotide i.e. NAD with Hydrogen). There are many complex reactions and inter-reactions which link these important chemicals. The majority of the different Vitamin Bs play a pivotal role in effective and relatively safe metabolism.

Coenzyme A is another chemical that has a Sulphur component which is extremely useful in the fight against cancer. The importance of Sulphur components cannot be understated. Sulphur is an essential element in all our body's cells. It is the seventh or eighth most abundant element in the human body by weight, being about as common as potassium, and in fact is more common than sodium or chlorine. The amino acids cysteine and methionine which are present in plant and animal proteins contain the most Sulphur. Sulphur bonds strongly with itself creating disulphide bonds and these bonds play a key role in protein synthesis and structure. The two vitamins biotin and thiamine also contain Sulphur. Sulphur containing chemicals play a significant role in the so-called redox reactions necessary in metabolism.

Coenzyme A is made by the body in a range of ways but the easiest way to help your body create sufficient to help the Krebs Cycle is by taking sufficient Vitamin B-5 and by making sure you eat a varied protein diet that will allow your body to make cysteine and methionine which are amino acids. There are a wide range of food which you can eat that contain cysteine or its precursor but egg white, sesame seed flour, chicken, pork soy protein, brazil nut, onions, red peppers, garlic, oat and wheat-based foodstuffs contain high levels.

Cysteine has many varied and interesting uses within the body. It has been used by some to help combat the effects of a hangover. It is believed that this is effective due to cysteine's involvement in the conversion of acetaldehyde (a toxic waste product of alcohol metabolism) within the liver to a non-toxic waste product. Increased amounts of cysteine and Vitamin B-1 (thiamine) appear from animal studies at least to significantly increase the liver's performance in combating acetaldehyde. Following this link anything that improves the liver's function in managing toxins is worth considering in your fight against cancer. Vitamin B-1's scientific name is thiamine which stems from its important thio or Sulphur content. Vitamin B-1 is highly utilized by nerve cells especially and a shortage in your diet leads to serious complications such as "beriberi". The Recommended Dietary Allowance RDA is very low and based on the requirement for normal existence. Studies have shown that significantly higher levels can be taken safely for normal adults. In helping the liver function it is a highly important chemical in fighting cancer and so it is essential that at least the recommended daily amount (RDA) of vitamin B-1 is taken. There are no known significant toxic side-effects from too much vitamin B-1 intake in normal healthy adults noted so many people often taken at least twice this amount for the duration of their treatment and fight against cancer i.e. for at least 60 days but obviously this is a personal choice which should definitely be made in consultation with your doctor.

NADH is a metabolically active form of Vitamin B3 (niacin). In pharmacological doses, niacin has been proven to reverse atherosclerosis by reducing total cholesterol but also increasing high-density lipoprotein (HDL). This is believed to reduce the likelihood of thrombosis. NADH is essential for the production of cellular energy (ATP) from glucose and fat. Simplistically the more NADH a cell has available, the more energy it has available to operate with optimal efficiency, but there are both limits to what the body can use and which are safe. Nicotinamide Adenine Dinucleotide, NAD is the oxidated form of NADH and is also a coenzyme found in all human cells. Nucleotides are chemicals, which are important in cell metabolism but also when combined make up components of DNA. NAD can also be made by the body from the amino acids tryptophan and aspartic acid, which are common in a range of protein-based foods such as eggs, meat, fish, soy beans, nuts, wheat etc. Aspartic acid is a non-essential amino acid and so the body can synthesize it if necessary. Tryptophan is an essential amino acid to be eaten as the human body cannot synthesize it (see below). NADH is not just involved in cell metabolism but it is also directly involved in chemical reactions relating to the immune system, the nerve system (neurotransmission) and the repair of DNA. Not surprisingly then this is a highly important chemical in fighting cancer and so it is essential that at least the recommended daily amount (RDA) of vitamin B-3 is taken. There are toxic side-effects from too much vitamin B-3 intake in normal healthy adults so intake should be controlled but many people often taken twice this amount for the duration of their treatment and fight against cancer i.e. for at least 60 days but obviously this is a personal choice which should definitely be made in consultation with your doctor.

If the body is run down or fighting infection, then it can react differently to vitamins during an inflammatory phase. A scientific research study of nearly 900 older adults showed that low Vitamin B6 levels were linked to higher C-Reactive Protein levels. In this study the plasma levels of pyridoxal 5-phosphate (PLP) was also checked. A low circulating level of vitamin B_6 has been noted as a risk factor for cardiovascular diseases. Vitamin B6 is a water-soluble vitamin and is part of the B complex group. Several forms of the vitamin are known, but PLP is the active form and is a cofactor in many important chemical reactions involving protein metabolism. PLP is also an essential part of two important enzymes. Low vitamin B_6 levels will mean decreased activity of these enzymes.

Pyridoxine has a role in preventing heart disease. Without enough pyridoxine, a compound called homocysteine builds up in the body. Homocysteine damages blood vessel linings, setting the stage for plaque build-up when the body tries to heal the damage. Vitamin B_6 prevents this build-up, thereby reducing the risk of heart attack. Pyridoxine lowers blood pressure and blood cholesterol levels and keeps blood platelets from sticking together.

Research has shown that vitamin B_6 intake and pyridoxal PLP levels are inversely related to the risk of cancer of the colon. Although the correlation with vitamin B_6 intake was moderate, there was a significant link with PLP levels where the risk of colon cancer was nearly decreased in half.

BIOTIN – a.k.a. vitamin B7
Biotin is necessary for cell growth, the production of fatty acids, and the metabolism of fats and proteins. It is involved in the citric acid cycle, which is the reaction where energy is released via aerobic respiration. Biotin not only is involved in various metabolic reactions but also helps to move carbon dioxide.

Tryptophan
Tryptophan is one of the standard essential amino acids needed by the body as it can't be made by humans. Luckily it is present in a wide range of foodstuffs and so as long as you have a well-balanced diet you are not likely to be short of it. However during cancer your body's functioning is probably less than 100% and so additional intake or supplements may not be a bad idea. As you would expect for an amino acid it is high in protein-based foods especially egg white, fish and soy beans but also the majority of meats etc. Many people find that increases in these foods or tryptophan supplements aid getting a good night's sleep. This is a healthy additional benefit which might be useful in your fight against cancer. It is believed that these increased tryptophan levels lead in turn to increased secretion levels of serotonin and melatonin within the brain from the pineal gland. These chemicals are your brain's way of helping to induce sleep during darkness, which is why most people naturally sleep at night when there is generally no or low levels of light. It is no surprise to me that there is lots of research to show that most humans are happier and less

likely to be irritable or depressed if they have sufficient sleep. From the point of view of fighting cancer you need your body giving its peak physiological performance if it is to deal with the cancer and any treatments. It will be better placed to achieve this with sufficient sleep.

In general all B vitamins need to be taken at sufficient levels (RDA as a minimum) to help the body maintain and increase metabolism, help improve the body's immune system, help maintain healthy red blood cells, help maintain nerve function and aid natural cell activity such as growth. They also help maintain good liver and pancreas function which is essential to aid your fight against cancer. Some deficiencies of B vitamins have been linked to cancers especially Vitamin B-12. You only need a small amount of vitamin B-12 each day and generally if you eat a healthy balanced diet and don't have a condition that affects your absorption of vitamin B-12 (like anaemia) you're unlikely to need supplements and generally those B vitamins absorbed from food are preferred. If you eat a vegan diet, it can be difficult for you to get enough vitamin B-12 because it isn't found in any vegetable matter (including grains). Vitamin B-12 is in high levels in meat, eggs and cheese.

Many breakfast cereals have added B vitamins which help you to maintain your intake. Luckily a good varied diet which includes eggs and meat usually means you will get sufficient B vitamins but taking supplements is a good idea as most B vitamins need regular intake as any excess is excreted in your urine. This means that on the whole it is hard for you to have toxic amounts of B vitamins. Vitamins B-3, B-6, B-9, B-7 & B12 have mild side-effects if taken to excess.

According to the Institute of Medicine Food and Nutrition Board, USA a maximum daily amount of 35 mg/day for vitamin B-3 should not be exceeded as you may suffer nausea, flushing and itchy skin etc. Of interest however is that doctors often prescribe recommended doses up to 2000 mg. per day of slow-release niacin for patients with arterial plaques and high lipid levels. Once again an attempt to control an inflammatory problem could be useful in helping you fight your cancer. The interaction with other treatments must be considered carefully especially at these high levels. According to the Institute of Medicine Food and Nutrition Board, USA a maximum daily amount of 100 mg/day for vitamin B-6 should not be exceeded as you may suffer from nerve side-effects. According to the Institute of Medicine Food and Nutrition Board, USA a maximum daily amount of 1 mg/day for vitamin B-9 should not be exceeded as you may hide a vitamin B-12 deficiency which would be serious.

Recommended Dietary/Daily Allowance
The Recommended Dietary Allowance (RDA) system was originally devised by scientists during World War II as a means of helping assess the food needs of soldiers who were practically all male at that time. There have been several updates since then for it to guide the public and not just the armed forces. In 1997 the term was re-named to be a daily value so is often called the RDI (Reference Daily Intake). The RDI is an estimate of the level required by an average, healthy person to avoid showing signs of deficiency. With any average estimate there is degree of unsuitability for a specific adult male or female. It is fair to say that a healthy you will have your own individual daily need which will be different from the RDI as it is impossible for the stated RDI to be perfect for everyone. It is far from perfect but it is good starting point. The RDI in theory states the minimum level of a nutrient needed to stay healthy. This intake is not the same thing as how much the body actually uses, since the body is not a perfect machine and

generally absorbs less of a particular nutrient than is actually in the food. Many scientists feel that the RDI levels maybe significantly dated especially regarding antioxidant levels which many convincingly argue should be up to 400% higher. The RDI need for an active healthy 18 year old is likely to be different to an inactive healthy 90 year old and so on. The point I am trying to make is that it is far from an exact science such that a person with cancer is likely to have a very different need to the average healthy adult and that these recommended levels should be considered a starting point for your decisions regarding your own intake.

Well I think you will agree there is a lot to take in this chapter, much of which will also help you understand the next chapter. In summary of this chapter you want to limit the excess production of natural toxins (ROS) and you want to help every cell in your body work efficiently. This can be achieved by ensuring that your body has ready access to all the B vitamins and certain proteins. A balanced and varied diet is important which could include egg white or egg white powder and some meat especially chicken is a good start. Next are your jobs to do and tick off.

Jobs To Do

1. Buy a juicer and make fresh vegetable/fruit juices/smoothies every day. See the internet for great recipes
2. Have eggs as part of your diet and enjoy marmite on toast regularly to aid vitamin and sulphur intake.
3. Have fish at least twice a week
4. Try liver and/or chicken at least once a week
5. If not keen on meat eat a lot of nuts (especially brazil and walnuts), chick peas, beans and lentils
6. Take at the very least the Recommended Dietary Allowance (RDA i.e. "Recommended Daily Amount") of all your Vitamin Bs (B-1, B-2, B-3, B-5, B-6, B-7, B-9, B-12) for a short period of time as a kick start for their recuperation and fight against cancer i.e. for at least 2 weeks.

AS PREVIOUSLY STATED NUMEROUS TIMES THIS IS A PERSONAL CHOICE WHICH SHOULD BE MADE IN CONSULTATION WITH YOUR DOCTOR.

Chapter 8: Oxidative Stress & Enzymes

Oxidative Stress is a term often used to explain when the natural balance (homeostasis) of the body is out of balance. It should be remembered that oxidation and strong oxidant production is a normal part of human physiology and is highly important part of normal cell metabolism. Oxidative stress is a condition where more strong oxidants are produced than can be dealt with ("scavenged").

Most oxidative damage in cells takes place due to potential toxic chemicals known as Reactive Oxygen Species (ROS). The healthy balance of necessary oxidants and toxic oxidants is maintained by the body in part by its use of antioxidants under normal healthy operating conditions. This battle is like the constant battle between good and evil or matter and anti-matter in that it is rare that the balance is perfect and one of the two is usually on top. A significant amount of ROS occur in humans during healthy life due to the leakage of activated oxygen from mitochondria during oxidative phosphorylation. Other organisms such as bacteria within the body are also producers of ROS but to a lesser degree. ROS are produced by a wide variety of the human body's enzymes under normal conditions. ROS play important roles in cell signaling and so to maintain a natural healthy balance the human body must manage the "creation" and "destruction" of ROS.

Most ROS are produced at a low level by normal cellular metabolism and the cell damage they manage to cause is continually repaired. ROS are potentially highly toxic molecules in large concentrations. Unfortunately, when oxidative stress levels are high and maintained then repair cannot occur quickly enough before long term cell damage is caused. This oxidative damage can affect a specific molecule, entire cell, area or even the whole organ. The most significant cell damage regarding your fight against cancer is that done to DNA. Oxidative damage can include single-strand breaks, modification of base pairs, and cross-links between strands of DNA. If the DNA repair mechanisms are unable to fix the damage, the damaged DNA may contain various mutations that can affect cellular function, and in some cases this leads to carcinogenesis.

Excess levels of ROS are linked to many diseases including neurodegenerative diseases (such as Parkinson's & Alzheimer's), cataracts, atherosclerosis, diabetes and heart disease as well as in the aging process itself. Exposure to ROS over time leads to damaged DNA and the modification of proteins and other molecules. In a healthy adult it has been estimated that the body's cells have their DNA assaulted by ROS about 10,000 times per day clearly with the passage of time and a repair system that is not perfect (human) a degradation process is inevitable commonly known as aging. It has been shown in many animal studies that by limiting diet to its basic needs (i.e. not over-eating) that signs of degradation (aging) are less and healthy lifespan is expanded. These studies have linked the reduced oxidative stress that a limited diet creates as a possible significant factor.

Oxidative stress occurs when there is increased production of ROS or a significant decrease in the antioxidant defenses. It is important to re-iterate that oxidative damage by excessive ROS can be limited or even prevented by anti-oxidants. The human body itself produces and contains anti-oxidants to prevent the harmful effects of ROS if the daily diet is good. There are loads of antioxidants, some which are edible and some which the body needs to make (synthesize). One very important one which the body needs to make for example is glutathione (GSH). Raising GSH levels through direct supplementation of glutathione is difficult. Research suggests that glutathione taken orally is not well absorbed by the gut. Even when very large doses are given orally it has not been demonstrated clinically to have a significant impact. Glutathione (GSH) improves liver detoxification by combining with toxins and limiting their toxic effects as well as making them easier to excrete thus glutathione may be helpful in the treatment of liver disease, along with many other illnesses and toxic conditions. GSH helps cleanse the body of oxidative toxic by-products such as hydrogen peroxide and thus helps to protect the mitochondria (the cell's energy production unit), DNA and the cell membrane from damage.

Glutathione (GSH) is a very common chemical in most living organisms including humans. It is the most common thiol (carbon-based chemical containing sulphur group) found in cells. Glutathione is made from three amino acids cysteine, glutamic acid, and glycine. The amino acid cysteine is considered the limiting factor in most diets as the other two amino acids are readily available in most balanced diets. So if you are wishing to assist your body's natural synthesis of Glutathione it is a good idea to ensure you eat a fair supply of cysteine which is found in sufficient quantities in high protein foods (such as chicken, eggs, milk, cottage cheese and yoghurt). Cyanohydroxybutene, a chemical found in broccoli, cauliflower, Brussels sprouts and cabbage, is also thought to increase glutathione levels. Certain herbs like cinnamon and Turmeric have chemicals that can help to maintain good levels of glutathione too. Brazil nuts contain a high amount of selenium which can increase glutathione levels. Other vegetable foodstuffs considered good at assisting in raising glutathione levels are red peppers, onions, garlic, oats, lentils and wheat germ. All human cells are able to synthesize glutathione to some degree but the majority is synthesized by the liver. This is yet another major reason for maintain liver health during your fight against cancer.

Although excessive sun exposure is not advised regular daily exposure especially in people of the northern hemisphere can be extremely beneficial in maintaining **Vitamin D** levels. Vitamin D increases glutathione levels generally but especially in the brain and is directly linked to the body's natural glutathione production. The amount of activated vitamin D in the brain is tied to how much vitamin D3 one has, either ingested through supplements or created in the skin via sun exposure. This suggests taking vitamin D3 supplements and/or getting adequate sensible sun exposure boosts glutathione production.

There is a GSH precursor called **N-acetylcysteine** or NAC for short. NAC is the most commonly available in food precursor other supplements and whey protein have also been shown to increase GSH levels. Aging bodies can easily convert NAC into the eye-protecting antioxidant glutathione, defending the eye from harmful free radicals. These two key ingredients reduce oxidative damage to retinal cells and thus help protect the eye. NAC is available both as a prescribed drug but also as a generic supplement, but is found in sufficient levels in many protein-based foods such as chicken, cheese, eggs and sunflower seeds.

Another well-known liver tonic from history is the milk thistle and its seeds and these have been shown to increase GSH levels. When well, body GSH levels are regulated by negative feedback pathways and so there are limits to the benefits of taking excessive amounts of precursors. However when you are unwell GSH levels have been noted as low in cases of oxidative stress and thus a wide range of pathologies such as cancer and malnutrition especially. Due to the potential damage of free radicals to organs including the brain low GSH levels have been noted in patients with Alzheimer's disease and bipolar depressive disorders.

Regarding cancer, GSH has both protective and regenerative activities. It is crucial in the removal and detoxification of carcinogens, and alterations in this pathway, can have a profound effect on cell survival. However, by conferring resistance to a number of chemotherapeutic drugs, elevated levels of glutathione in tumour cells are able to protect such cells in bone marrow, breast, colon, larynx and lung cancers. Although glutathione has shown success in reducing cancer growth in the lab and in animal studies, there are limited reported trials in humans appear to be reported as discussed earlier possibly to body processes impacting directly on the GSH levels.

It seems that today unfortunately in the western world at least that many of us are probably at an abnormally high level of oxidative stress risk primarily due to our processed and meat-based diets and oxidant toxic environments as discussed earlier, which could explain to some degree the increased risk and incidence of cancer and other diseases.

Managing Oxidative Stress with Antioxidant Enzymes

The Odd SODs

Superoxide is one of the main Reactive Oxygen Species (ROS) created in a human cell by the mitochondria. The human body controls this potentially dangerous chemical type by a range of enzymes known as the Super Oxide Dismutases or more affectionately abbreviated to the SODs. The SODs manage at speed the breakdown of superoxide. SODs are therefore an important part in every cell's protection from oxidative damage especially to the DNA structures in the cell's nucleus. The SODs play a key role in all cells' antioxidant defense. There are 3 general types of SODs categorized as SOD1, SOD2 & SOD3s. The SOD enzymes are complex proteins which contain metals within them (Copper, Zinc and Manganese).

SOD1 contains Copper & Zinc and is found within the general human cell structure.
SOD2 contains **Manganese** and is found within the mitochondria of the human cell.
SOD3 contains Copper & Zinc and is found outside the human cell.

A lot of research into SODs has taken place over the last 30 odd years and low levels in animal studies have yielded interesting results. For example when mice had no ability to make SOD1 they suffered a range of illness including many so-called inflammatory diseases such as cataracts and cancer. Mice that had no ability to make SOD2 died within days of birth due to extreme oxidative stress and damage. Mice that had no ability to make SOD3 were less impacted but still had a significantly shorter lifespan than normal mice.

SODs have been used to improve skin appearance by limiting oxidative damage and limiting fibrosis (formation of scar tissue). SOD therapy has been used to try and limit the fibrosis which often occurs following radiation particularly of the breast

Other studies have linked reduced SOD levels to other neural and inflammatory conditions including Crohn's Disease, high blood pressure, colon inflammation and increased cancer risk. Increased SOD levels have been seen to limit leucocyte and endothelial adhesions and so yet again a link with inflammatory problems, their control and cancer.

In short all SODs are present in or around the cell so are obviously well placed for their specific roles but the often called SOD2 enzyme is right at the centre of the oxidation action being present within the mitochondria. To me these are the most important in limiting excessive oxidative stress. Clearly it is important to have your dietary intake of all trace metals (especially Iron, Copper, Zinc, and Manganese) but due to SOD2 enzymes location and their major impact I would focus on the manganese component especially as this an essential component of the SOD-2 enzyme.

There are oral supplements available which report to increase SOD levels within the body but due to the digestive system only a small percentage of the SOD is directly available to the body. This concept is often referred to as the bio-availability factor of a supplement. It occurs because a significant amount of the supplement has been broken down to its component parts by the digestive system and these component parts (other chemicals) can be used for other purposes. Many have attempted to overcome this by coating the supplement and/or combining it with other chemicals. Different types of supplement have undergone a number of scientific studies and some appear to retain bioavailability following digestion. The SOD is obtained from **cantaloupe melons** (melons with orange flesh inside) which are high in SOD. Clearly by increasing your consumption of cantaloupe melons you could increase very slightly your SOD levels. Eating the melon fresh also gives the added benefits of other polyphenols and Vitamin C.

Glutathione Antioxidant Enzymes
The human body produces a number of other antioxidant enzymes apart from the SODs. The most significant other ones which also help convert ROS in the fight against oxidative damage are considered to be catalase, glutathione peroxidase and glutathione reductase.

Catalase is another enzyme which is useful in managing oxidative stress and luckily is fairly common being found in all human cells, where it catalyzes (speeds up) detoxification. It is a complex protein with **iron** complexes present. Catalase is highly useful in managing ROS following on from the action of SODs. In particular catalase helps with the further superoxide breakdown from hydrogen peroxide to water and oxygen. It is an enzyme involved in the breakdown of a range of toxins including alcohol. Not surprisingly due to its detoxification role it is found in high concentrations in the liver. Catalase is a very busy and effective enzyme in that just one molecule can help change up to approximately 40 million molecules of hydrogen peroxide to water and oxygen in a second. It is a strange enzyme and little understood physiologically.

For example in mice bred to have no catalase they were found to survive relatively normally. However it has been noted that there is an increased risk of diabetes in people with very low levels of catalase. Also of relevance and interest is that there is up to one hundred times more catalase present in normal cells than cancer cells which seem to have a major deficiency of this enzyme. It has been found that glutathione enzymes become more active when levels of catalase are low. This is again another link to an inflammatory disease potentially caused by oxidative damage. Catalase is present in practically every foodstuff and is substantially broken down so that supplements are not probably beneficial. Many people though decide to increase their intake of certain **foods high in catalase such as beef liver, potatoes, avocados, bananas, leeks, onions, radishes, carrots, spinach, parsnips, and red cabbage**. These foodstuffs are also high in other important nutrients and so are helpful to improve your cancer-fighting diet. The majority, apart from maybe avocados and the liver which are high in fat, can be consumed in high amounts without any major side effects.

Glutathione peroxidase is like catalase in that it is another group of enzymes which is useful in managing oxidative stress and luckily is fairly common being found in and around all human cells, where it also manages ROS and catalyzes (speeds up) the detoxification of hydrogen peroxide to water. Glutathione peroxidase has many physiological functions including DNA repair, metabolism of toxins and carcinogens and support of the immune system. Glutathione peroxidase is an enzyme which is considered a member of the selenoprotein family. Its importance and action in humans is not fully understood yet. However glutathione peroxidase plays an important role in managing oxidative damage by catalyzing the reduction hydro peroxides. It does this by using glutathione as the reducing chemical. It is essential to ensure that your body has sufficient Selenium to manufacture glutathione peroxidase and possible during your fight against cancer to briefly increase your Selenium intake for a period of time. This is because of the key role glutathione peroxidase plays in maintaining the healthy structure of all membranes (both cellular and intracellular membranes).

Research into oxidative damage is wide-ranging even to the point of using carcinogenic compounds on animals and measuring the damage caused by toxins such as Mercury. Oxidative stress is controlled and less chromosomal damage is noted when there are increased levels of oxidized glutathione and glutathione peroxidase found in the liver and brain. Maintaining glutathione levels using its associated enzymes is an essential part of the body's natural protection from either self-made or external toxins. Healthy levels of Glutathione are essential in managing the damage caused blood sugars combining with proteins or fats. This chemical reaction of sugars, glycation, can create many problems for the body. Glycation is increased in people suffering from diabetes and can cause many of the problems related to diabetes such as interfering with RBCs' haemoglobin and causing them to be less efficient in delivering oxygen and interfering with proteins in the eye thus affecting sight. Glycation has also been implicated in other diseases of the kidney, pancreas, nervous system and bone system. It has been linked to chronic inflammatory and so-called age-related diseases such heart disease, Alzheimer's disease and cancer. One of the recurring links of many of these varied diseases is that of low and poorly maintained glutathione levels. It is not to say that this is a simple link with a clear cause and effect, but many studies have shown that increased glutathione levels and its associated enzyme levels have led to improvements in a range of diseases and their symptoms. This is very important information for you to be aware in your fight against cancer.

Glutathione Reductase (GR) is another enzyme that is involved in detoxification. It regenerates glutathione that is used as a hydrogen donor by glutathione peroxidase during the detoxification of hydrogen peroxide. The activity of GR is used as a biochemical marker for oxidative stress. Glutathione reductase is a flavoprotein that is required for the conversion of oxidized glutathione to reduced glutathione (GSH). At the same time, it oxidizes nicotinamide adenine dinucleotide phosphate (NADPH). Flavoproteins are proteins which contain a chemical derivative (nucleic acid) of riboflavin (**Vitamin B2**). This is another important reason to maintain at least the recommended dietary allowance of this vitamin and as previously stated to possible increase intake above this during times when fighting disease which can increase ROS such as cancer. It is important to be aware that increased levels of Vitamin B2 intake leads to your urine being much more yellow in colour as significant excess is excreted from the body. GR is an exceptionally common enzyme and is essential for the regulation of reduced glutathione (GSH) levels. Reduced glutathione plays an important role in Redox reactions and also in the detoxification of peroxides. Peroxides are potentially dangerous chemicals which are made in very large quantities by cells during diseases which are linked to inflammation. GR as a consequence is directly linked to chemical reactions involving glutathione peroxidase.

Low levels of GR can lead to damage to Red Blood Cells membranes and eventual rupture which obviously is not going to help you in your fight against cancer. Generally your body's natural homeostasis ability means that as long as the right nutrients are received, that it adapts to the fluctuations naturally on a demand basis. For example it has been found that high levels of glutathione reductase have been found in the RBCs of people suffering from the inflammatory process linked to their rheumatoid arthritis as their bodies try to manage the process.

Glutathione-S-Transferase (GST) is another family of enzymes that are involved in detoxification. This superfamily of enzymes is important in cell defense processes. These enzymes link reduced glutathione to many toxic compounds, including chemotherapy drugs. GST focuses on the detoxification of carcinogenic chemicals introduced to the body rather than those made by the body as a by-product. Turmeric which is well known for its health benefits by Indians is a spice which not only contains Curcumin also appears to contain GST. Therefore Turmeric is being extensively researched regarding its antioxidant, anti-inflammatory and anti-cancer cell behaviour.

The body's ability to produce these enzymes appears to decrease with age. During normal stages of cell multiplication (normal growth) the body has high levels of these enzymes to manage the oxidative stress and limit damage. Obviously during childhood there is a maximum growth spurt and therefore the body has significantly higher levels of these enzymes. It appears that with time and less growth the body's ability to produce these enzymes is reduced. Clearly a diet full of the appropriate pre-cursors is a good way to maintain healthy levels of production. Eating a healthy diet full of raw foods, fruits, nuts, vegetables, proteins, herbs and spices, all help keep your Glutathione S-Transferase enzymes functioning optimally.

Supplements of these enzymes are available and have been researched. However the human body will break a fair percentage down during digestion so that absorption of these enzymes is likely to be limited at best. Supplementing with the components the body requires to make these enzymes may be more effective. These include the minerals manganese, zinc and copper for SOD and selenium for glutathione peroxidase.

In addition to SOD, glutathione peroxidase and catalase, many vitamins and minerals are effective antioxidants in their own right, such as vitamin E, vitamin C, lutein, lycopene, vitamin B2, coenzyme Q10, and cysteine (an amino acid). Herbs, such as grape seed, bilberry, turmeric (curcumin), ginkgo, milk thistle and green tea also contain powerful antioxidant compounds. Many experts believe that the best way to provide the body with the most complete protection against free radicals is to consume a large variety of antioxidants.

Key transition metals such as **Copper, Zinc, Manganese, Iron & Selenium** are important in the production of ROS. They are often involved in redox reactions and can lead to the production of free radicals and ROS. The majority of phase 1 enzymes that we talked about earlier have a transition metal within them and can produce ROS.

Most transition metals except Zinc are considered radicals as they have unpaired electrons. They can convert some of the less reactive oxidants into highly reactive free radicals or ROS. In the body Copper and Iron are the most common and key chemicals for important chemical reactions. These reactions involve metal ions which are bound to the surface of proteins, DNA, and other large molecules. These metal ions can still be involved in redox reactions whereas other transition metals that are imbedded in proteins such as cytochromes are not able to be involved in redox reactions.

The severity of damage caused by ROS is often linked to its location of production. With regards to cancer primarily we are concerned about any possible damage or mutation caused to the DNA so due to transition metals not being in a free state in the human body but usually bonded or imbedded to a site it means that ROS are more likely to react at specific location rather than in a more random way due to its unpaired electrons. This obviously leads to the same location being "hit" repeatedly by ROS more that it would if it were truly random which can lead to serious and unrepairable breaks to the DNA helix.

As already stated selenium is a part of the enzyme glutathione peroxidase and this knowledge has helped explain the importance of both selenium and vitamin E. Many studies infer a benefit of reduced prostatic cancer by using selenium and Vitamin E supplements. This has not been backed by all researchers with some large scale studies even showing no benefit.

Selenium is of key importance in your fight against cancer and so warrants further discussion. Interestingly the importance of selenium in managing oxidative damage is almost as old as the earth we understand to be the living planet. It is estimated that over three billion years ago blue-green algae were the first living cells to produce the poisonous product we know as oxygen in the atmosphere by photosynthesis. These algae would have been in danger of quickly killing themselves were it not for the antioxidant system which works by the interaction of selenium, iodine and peroxidase enzymes. It is widely known that seaweeds contain high levels of selenium and iodine and that many people around the world eat seaweed as a source of these important trace minerals. **Iodide** also helps manage reactive oxygen species (ROS) in humans. The importance of iodine in the diet cannot be underestimated either, apart from its well-known role in the hormone thyroxine which regulates metabolism, natural development and growth it is also present in significant amounts in other forms in the breasts, eyes, gastric mucosa, the cervix, and salivary glands. The thymus gland also has high levels of iodine present which would tend to link iodine's importance to immune system as the thymus gland produces white blood cells (aka "T-cells").

Biologically selenium was first noted in the early twentieth century to be toxic to cows that consumed plants with a high selenium content. Selenium is an essential trace element for humans to remain healthy which is especially true in cases of low levels of Vitamin E. The liver can suffer severely if both these are absent or extremely low in the diet at the same time. It was not until the late 1970's that more extensive studies on the importance of selenium in the human diet took place. In plants selenium is found in a complex chemical selenomethionine and generally, while the most in animal foods selenium is found in a complex chemical is selenocysteine. Humans tend to absorb selenium from the duodenum, which is the section of the digestive tract directly after the stomach. It appears that the body absorbs Selenium better from plant foodstuffs in the form of selenomethionine. There is limited agreement but it appears that wheat, cow's kidneys and Brazil Nuts offer the best source of selenium to the body in that order. There is little agreement it seems on how the human body regulates its intake of Selenium or transports it around the body. The recommended daily allowance is 70mcg for men and 55mcg for women. When fighting cancer many people have found to get significant benefits over a short period that up to 600mcg can be taken. Many studies have found that higher levels of Selenium than the recommended daily allowance has resulted in very significantly lower deaths due to cancer. There is also evidence selenium can help during chemotherapy treatment by improving the treatment's effectiveness and by, reducing the toxicity of certain chemotherapeutic drugs. Lab studies have shown that certain chemotherapeutic drugs are more effective at killing cancer cells when selenium is present. Selenium has also been shown to act by itself by directly causing cell death in cancer cells. Selenium has been seen to be effective in helping in the fight against very many different cancers. It has also been proved to helpful in managing many other inflammatory diseases by managing adhesions and cholesterol in general. Its anti-inflammatory action is improved when combined with Vitamin E. Its interaction with iodine and thyroxine helps ensure a good metabolism and its activating role helps maintain a healthy immune system.

Having low levels of Selenium is rare if you eat a balanced diet. As stated before too much selenium is toxic so use a fair degree of common sense when deciding how much you will take and over what period. Some of the side effects include nausea and vomiting, hair loss and altered mental state such as depression and increased anxiety. The consumption of selenium, though necessary, is dangerous if not monitored properly. The human body needs only about 400 micrograms of selenium per day. The symptoms of selenium poisoning are commonly hair loss and brittleness of the finger nails and toe nails.

All this information should indicate that it is probably wise to get your selenium uptake from Brazil Nuts and not to take excessively high levels of Selenium supplements due to its potentially toxic capabilities.

Manganese is a particularly important trace element for your body as it has a role in general absorption, enzyme function, brain function, the healing function, and healthy bones development. If levels of Manganese are very low in the body this can result in bone and fertility problems. The RDA for Manganese is 2mg but during illness as previous stated individual needs maybe greater.

Many foodstuffs have Manganese present in fair amounts but the winners, weight for weight, are Ground Cloves & Saffron (see earlier chapter). Other good sources of Manganese include **hazelnuts, pinenuts, sunflower seeds, flax seeds, sesame seeds, wheat germ and wheat bran**. More enjoyable to most people is chocolate which contains a fair amount of Manganese especially dark chocolate ideally unsweetened but even a small increase in Manganese is better than none. Another spice that is high in Manganese is chilli powder so why not have a hot curry instead with cloves, pinenuts, sunflower seeds and chilli. Manganese does help in antioxidant protection in the form of Manganese Super Oxide Dismutase (MnSOD). Manganese has also been noted to be deficient in people with certain types of baldness and so maybe useful in helping hair regrowth after chemotherapy induced loss. However be very aware that excessive levels of manganese are toxic and so supplements should be approached with care.

Body Management of Oxidative Stress - Phase 1 and Phase 2 Enzymes pre-cursors

All cells are involved in the homeostasis necessary to keep oxidative stress under control and limit any subsequent oxidative damage caused by toxic chemicals. However some are specifically designed for this fight against toxic chemicals. The cells of the liver are highly organized and large in number. The liver is the first organ that is served by the blood system after the blood has received nutrients from the gut and so is well placed to detoxify the blood and thus protect other "weaker" organs from damage. Although the liver is the detox king we should not underestimate the important detox job done by the epithelial cells of the gut first as well as the contribution made by the epithelial cells of the kidneys, lungs and skin. All these must be working as well as possible if improvements in our fight against cancer are to be made.

Cells in the liver are the most active in dealing with toxins although every cell has a limited ability to manage toxins but liver cells have the highest concentrations of these enzymes. Also important in this toxic waste management are the epithelial cells of the kidney, gut, lungs and skin. Clearly all these are important but a healthy working liver is essential in this toxic waste management.

The body often removes or converts toxins (harmful chemicals) within the body by the use of enzymes, which help convert complex toxins into water-soluble chemicals which can be excreted from the body primarily urine, sweat and in the moisture present in the exhaled breath. That smell from someone who is suffering a hangover is a good example of toxic by-products being excreted from their sweat and breath. These enzymes are proving to be highly important for managing carcinogenic toxins, oxidative stress and therefore limiting oxidative damage. Substantial research has occurred regarding these enzymes especially the Phase 2 enzymes in particular in the fight against cancer.

Phase I enzyme in the cells called cytochrome P450 is one of the body's primary defences against toxic chemicals ingested with food. However, the induction of these enzymes to prevent damage by toxic foreign chemicals like drugs and pesticides also results in the production of oxidant by-products.

Phase I reactions are often oxidative reactions which involve cytochrome P450 enzymes (CYP), NADPH and oxygen, which can in themselves create toxic by-products which Phase II enzymes must detoxify further and make water-soluble. CYPs are many and varied but have are proteins with an iron and cysteine-based complex. CYPs are complex in their actions and interactions and so it is important to be aware that foodstuffs can interact in a range of ways for example grapefruit and starfruit and their juices have chemicals which inhibit the way certain CYPs act and so it is widely recommended by the medical profession to avoid them during certain chemotherapy. St John's Wort is another plant that is best avoided during your treatment and fight against cancer due to its wide ranging impact on a range of CYPs.

If we wish to give our bodies as good a chance as possible in the fight against cancer it is important that we minimize excessive oxidative stress as much as possible. Luckily we can use our knowledge of these phase 1 and phase 2 enzymes to ensure our diets provide significant nutrients for these enzymes to be made by our bodies in the right amounts. It is accepted that it is generally not a good idea to increase phase 1 enzymes as this can lead to the production of free radicals or carcinogenic chemicals. Phase 2 enzymes on the other hand are able to produce scavenging chemicals which should reduce oxidative stress significantly and therefore be our helpers in the fight against cancer. The enzymes themselves cannot be taken by mouth directly because our digestive system will naturally break them down and so if considering our diet and/or supplements which may help in the fight against cancer then pre-cursors need to be considered. Chemicals which help in the body's production of phase 2 enzymes we will call phase 2 enzyme pre-cursors and are well known in the area of diet management that can aid in the fight against cancer.

Many naturally occurring chemicals present in food such as polyphenols and isoflavoniods have been found to be excellent antioxidants and phase 2 enzyme precursors. I will briefly list some of the more widely researched phase 2 enzyme pre-cursors which have been seen to increase phase 2 enzyme production. Many animal research studies on inflammation and oxidative stress show that high intake of dietary phase 2 enzyme pre-cursors can help control many toxic impacts of ROS.

- **Krill Oil** has high levels of keto-carotenoid, tetraterpenoid, astaxanthin.
- **Soy and broad / fava beans** have high levels of the isoflavonoid, phytoestrogen, genistein.
- **Flaxseed (oil)** has high levels of phytoestrogen, enterolactone.
- **Kale** has high levels of the flavonol, kaempferol
- **Strawberries, raspberries and blackberries** have high levels of the polyphenolic ellagic acid.
- **Blueberries and cranberries** have high levels of proanthocyanidin
- **Turmeric** has high levels of curcumin

Sulforaphane was recently isolated from one variety of broccoli as the major and very potent inducer of phase 2 detoxification enzymes in murine hepatoma cells in culture. Since phase 2 enzyme induction is often associated with reduced susceptibility of animals and their cells to the toxic and neoplastic effects of carcinogens and other electrophiles, it is possible that this is likely for humans.

All of the above in numerous studies have been seen to have significant impact on tumours and cancer cells. A number of studies have shown that phase 2 enzyme pre-cursors interfere with a range of cancerous cells' growth with animals treated with curcumin and astaxanthin showing a marked decrease in cell proliferation and increase in apoptosis. Phytoestrogens have been researched in cell lines and cases of breast and prostate cancers. Curcumin and ellagic acid have also been seen to protect the non-cancerous body from the incidental radiation damage from radiotherapy. One study showed that using soy protein, rather than milk-based proteins, in the diet of the stroke-prone rats improved their lifespan. It is believed that this may be due to the powerful phase 2 enzyme inducer genistein.

Alpha-Lipoic Acid (ALA)

ALA is a complex chemical which can have pro-oxidant properties which are used during detoxification and also can have antioxidant properties especially when linked with vitamin C and E. ALA is widely available from a healthy balanced diet. Interestingly it is another important chemical containing two complexes with Sulphur in them. The two sulphur molecules are able to be used repeatedly in oxidation and reduction reactions. This helps ALA to work as a powerful antioxidant that can control is capable of directly terminating potentially dangerous free radicals (oxidants). ALA has also been shown to have impacts on gene expression and repair oxidative damage

ALA is an essential chemical component for important enzymes found in the mitochondria. As discussed earlier about oxidative stress and aging older and or poor functioning mitochondria are less effective and more likely to produce higher levels of ROS. It has been found in many studies that levels of ALA or chemicals directly linked with ALA levels are reduced in a range of diseases. It seems to have multiple uses within the body and so not only does it have impact within the mitochondria's use of glucose it also helps increase cellular glutathione and vitamin C and manage toxic metals.

ALA is able to reduce ROS and interact with a large number of potential toxins including Mercury and Potassium Cyanide. It also can help to reduce chemicals which are linked with inflammation and cell damage generally. It has been linked with good liver physiology and been used as part of a range of treatments for a range of diseases and problems such as coronary heart disease, Alzheimer's Disease, diabetes, lowering cholesterol, toxic liver damage and other diseases linked to inflammation, endothelial and metabolic dysfunction.

ALA is an omega-3 fatty acid and is found in rapeseed oil, flax seed, walnuts, soybean oil, pumpkin seed oil, seaweed, algae and grasses. **Freshly ground flax seeds** contain 40% ALA with the rest containing proteins, lignans and phyto-oestrogens, which can have a protective effect against prostate cancer.

In recent years, ALA is being researched in detail as an anticancer agent due to results obtained from anti-proliferation studies on cancerous cell-based models. Some studies have suggested that ALA induces natural cancer cell death which is a major problem with most active cancer cells not receiving their natural signal to die.

ALA has also been proved to induce protective genes involved in the prevention of carcinogenesis in cellular studies, although how ALA achieves this is unknown.

Although once again not a wonder drug it certainly is a highly influential chemical within the body. ALA is present in most foodstuffs but is slightly higher cow's liver and kidneys, broccoli and yeast. It is therefore probably necessary or useful if you have cancer to increase your intake of these foodstuffs to obtain sufficient ALA but for a short period (60 days) it seems better to have large supplements of this when fighting cancer the human body's ability to make this chemical may be significantly impaired or its need far greater. Clearly as always consult your oncologist before any major changes to your diet or supplements.

Many degenerative diseases of the cardiovascular system and the central nervous system become more common as we age. There are a number of reasons which are understood why this happens and most are related to oxidative stress and its negative impact on the functioning of mitochondria leading to increased superoxide levels, with decreased abilities to produce GSH. The unknown is whether an increase in intake of phase 2 enzyme inducers can slow the impacts of aging significantly in humans but at least in rats studies have shown with consummation of good levels of strawberries, blueberry and spinach that the onset of neuronal deterioration is slowed. It appears that there is significant data to indicate these potent phase 2 inducers can slow what is often thought of as the normal ageing process.

Melatonin

Melatonin is a hormone produced by the pineal gland and released into the blood stream. Its main function seems to be to set and regulate our biological clock. Melatonin is also known to support the immune system by enabling more effective production of cell-signaling proteins, cytokines and has been used in the treatment of immunosuppressed patients such as those suffering with cancer or cancer treatment and HIV.

Melatonin present in White Blood Cells seems to be linked to the cytokine called interleukin-2 which is made during an immune response to help with the production a specific type of T-lymphocytes which are

WBCs which are capable of killing cancer cells. Melatonin taken with Calcium seems to stimulate the immune system more effectively than by themselves.

Cholesterol plays many important roles within the body's biochemistry and function. All are important in healthy function of the body but its actions as a component of cell membranes and involvement in vitamin D and hormone production is of high relevance in the fight against cancer. Cholesterol in the body is both from the diet or made by the body (biosynthesized). It is important to ensure that you have a balanced diet which does not include excessive cholesterol to minimize the prospect of chronic inflammation, arterial plaque formation, gallstones, heart attacks and strokes to name a few. However just to confuse things in your fight against cancer cholesterol is very important in the production of the powerful natural steroidal anti-inflammatory, hydrocortisone, which is also called **cortisol**. This very powerful steroid hormone is made in the adrenal glands using cholesterol and involving cytochrome P450 enzyme system.

Cortisol has many complex actions on a whole range of different cells but of most importance is that it damps down the body's immune system and interferes with the release of inflammatory chemicals. It reduces histamine production. Unfortunately excess cortisol over time can have many serious toxic side effects. It is best to try to enable your body to maintain its natural healthy levels (homeostasis) by a range of natural means. Cortisol has a significant role to play in the fight against cancer such that it is used by oncologists as part of the traditional medicine "toolkit".

Fluctuations in levels of cortisol in the blood have been linked to stress fluctuations. The stress can be of both the mental and physical kind for example depression or infection. Excess stress leads to very high levels of cortisol which is detrimental. It could be one of the reasons why some people have found meditation and relaxation beneficial in their fight against cancer as it may help de-stress and therefore regulate cortisol levels. Of significant interest is that its level in your body fluctuates naturally with your body's natural cycle, such that the lowest levels are usually present in the middle of the night and the highest levels approximately at normal waking time. This has led people to link it to the formation of the powerful antioxidant, melatonin. Lots of good quality sleep in a fully dark room is probably going to help lower your stress levels and restore the natural balance of cortisol and melatonin in your blood if low which is probably of significant benefit in your fight against cancer.

More important in the fight against cancer is the fact that Melatonin is an extremely powerful antioxidant reacts directly with ROS. Melatonin is present in food (fruits and vegetables and especially rice) and made by the body. Its ability to manage ROS is considerable in fact studies involving both animals and humans have shown it to have highly radio protective and anti-carcinogenic qualities. It has been used by travelers for many years to aid jet-lag as it induces drowsiness. Clearly if you are intending to use it in your fight against cancer then be aware that driving or using dangerous equipment is not recommended and that you should take it before sleep. It has excellent mobility around the body in that it easily crosses cell membranes and the blood-brain barrier. This is very useful for helping in the fight against all cancers including brain cancer. It has been used in patients suffering from Alzheimer's and Parkinson's disease with some success. It appears due to its antioxidant properties have a significant impact on inflammatory diseases. There have been studies which have shown reduced death rate over the short term in those cancer sufferers using melatonin. Melatonin works on fighting cancer by limiting excessive cell multiplication but by also stimulating natural cell death and the replacement of cancer cells with normal cells. It interacts with genetic switching at a cellular level which seems to occur during the aging process to regulate the genetic switching occurring in the cells throughout the body which promotes the aging process. It has been noted that the body produces less melatonin with age and in part its levels seem to explain why teenagers like to sleep all the time and the elderly sleep less. It has been considered by some a possible elixir of youth due to experiments on animals showing that the aging process speeds up in those animals with their pineal glands removed and those with inserted young pineal glands have longer lifespans. This might be a little simplistic to extrapolate for humans but nonetheless Melatonin is a very exciting chemical with interesting properties which are very useful in the fight against cancer.

Melatonin has been shown to interfere with cancer cells growth by suppressing a cancer tumour's usage of linoleic acid which is of prime importance in cell signaling. Dietary melatonin supplementation linked with eye-mask supported melatonin production has significant potential in the fight against cancer. Dark bedrooms are well known to aid sleep but also promote melatonin production. There appears increased cancer in people who work at night and it has been proposed that this is due significantly reduced melatonin levels. It does not appear that eating foods that contain melatonin significantly increase levels of melatonin within the body this maybe because it is converted quickly by reactions with ROS and so increased sleep in darkness maybe the only way to increase your body's level of melatonin. The benefits of a good night's sleep can never be underestimated.

Coenzyme Q10

Coenzyme Q10 (CoQ10) is a really important antioxidant present in and around most cells with high levels in the mitochondria and particularly high in the heart and liver cells which are both highly active in terms of energy consumption. Coenzyme Q10 (CoQ10) is heavily involved in cellular respiration using oxygen to help convert glucose into ATP. It is an antioxidant coenzyme that exists in three different states which means it can perform different functions easily. It is a key part of all cells structure and in particular its internal membranes. Due to its involvement in energy production it appears that coenzyme Q10 plays an important role in improving the immune system. It achieves this by increasing antibody production and aiding White Blood Cells. This improvement in the immune system has been noted in cancer sufferers and those suffering from other inflammatory and chronic diseases. Interestingly it has been noted that many diabetics are often suffering from low levels of CoQ10.

CoQ10 is a lipid-soluble benzoquinone found in all tissues and membranes. CoQ10 is particularly high in the inner mitochondrial membrane, where it acts in oxidative phosphorylation. CoQ10 is made by the body and is an antioxidant which protects membrane phospholipids from lipid-peroxidation. It has been heavily researched with significant evidence of its protective functions in cardio-vascular diseases and cancer.

CoQ10 is found in blood and in all organs. Deficiencies can be due to recessive mutations, ageing-related oxidative stress and carcinogenesis processes. In fact many neurological disorders, diabetes, cancer and cardiovascular diseases have been associated with reduced CoQ10 levels.

The antioxidant nature of CoQ10 arises from its role in energy conversion the chemical is continually involved in redox reactions. It is involved in the repetitive cycle of reduction and oxidation through its different states. CoQ10 is directly involved in stopping lipid peroxidation by stopping the initial creation of lipid peroxyl radicals and reducing the powerful ROS, singlet oxygen and hydrogen peroxide. These reactions help to protect both important cell lipids and cell proteins from damage. This can help stop damage and mutation to DNA occurring. Compared to many other antioxidants CoQ10 is more effective because of both its position (within the cell and mitochondria) but also its ability to protect both lipids and proteins. It is also closely linked with other antioxidants such that they work far more effectively. This lipid protection function of CoQ10 also helps secure LDL within the blood and therefore helps limit the formation of plaques with the blood vessels which is of major help in managing atherosclerosis. CoQ10 is made in a similar way to cholesterol by the body and so researchers have seen natural levels of CoQ10 also reduced in people who are using statins and so many people are taking CoQ10 supplements to counteract this potentially highly negative impact. A healthy cardiovascular system can be considered an essential piece of armoury in your fight against cancer.

There have been many interesting cases and studies regarding cancer control and CoQ10 in general, but particularly in patients with breast cancer. Fish such as sardines are high in naturally occurring CoQ10 but some people prefer supplements. Some well-respected researchers and clinicians have reported major benefits to people fighting cancer with cases of significant regression of some cancers and reduction in spread in others following supplementary treatment with CoQ10. The benefits have been noticed over the long term as well as short term (e.g. 60 days) with very high doses being used.

It appears that the lipid-soluble antioxidants like CoQ10, lycopene, some Vitamin As & Es and phytoestrogens such as genistein are the most effective in the fight against cancer as they are able to pass through cell membranes effectively and get to the places where they can be most effective in helping the cell i.e. mainly protecting the cells' DNA and mitochondria. Unfortunately the water soluble antioxidants although extremely useful are not so able to achieve this movement across membranes. This means it is difficult for water soluble antioxidants to be so active within the cancer cell.

CoQ10 is lipid-soluble and not soluble in water and so is absorbed by the small intestine. Therefore to help ensure healthy absorption if taking it as a supplement then it is best taken with lipids (e.g. oil such as olive oil). Many researchers have seen reduced abilities in humans to make CoQ10 especially in people suffering from chronic inflammatory diseases and also older adults. It is possible if you are suffering from cancer that this reduced production ability is also the case and that if fighting cancer you will also have a higher need for managing oxidative stress. Very large doses for short periods (such as 60days) are not considered toxic but clearly as always you should seek medical advice and listen to your body.

CoQ10 is thought of by many as the most important antioxidant against hydrogen peroxide because hydrogen peroxide is able to move across membranes as well and so is a very dangerous chemical. The good news is due CoQ10's ability to cross membranes the body is more able to make effective use of supplementation and due to its lipid solubility it is less likely to be excreted quickly.

Jobs to Do

1. Review chapter with red pen and highlight foods which you can comfortably incorporate in your diet **e.g. Krill Oil, Soy, broad / fava beans, Flaxseed (oil), Kale Strawberries, raspberries, blackberries, blueberries and cranberries &** <u>Turmeric.</u>

2. Consider supplements with your doctor tablets including **CoQ10, manganese, iron, copper, zinc and selenium.**

3. Eat freshly ground flax seeds try in a smoothie or salad.

4. Consider your sleep quality and darkness and consider **melatonin** intake with Calcium supplements (melatonin is a powerful drug and needs
a doctor's prescription in UK.

AS PREVIOUSLY STATED NUMEROUS TIMES THIS IS A PERSONAL CHOICE WHICH SHOULD BE MADE IN CONSULTATION WITH YOUR DOCTOR.

Chapter 9: Aspirin & other anti-inflammatories

The use of Aspirin in the long term care of heart disease and stroke is well known and Aspirin is widely used for its preventative benefits. Aspirin is a complex chemical when in the human body as it has a range of interactions far wider than just reducing blood platelet formation, which it is widely known for. These other interactions include a wide range of anti-inflammatory and protective impacts some of which will be explained in more detail.

Aspirin is truly a medicine of the ancients. Hippocrates used willow leaves, which contain high levels of Acetylsalicylic acid, to relieve inflammation linked to many illnesses in ancient Greece. From the bark of a willow tree in England in 1763 Rev. Edmund Stone improved aspirin understanding from ancient remedy to a drug by isolating salicin. Salicin is the glycoside of salicylic acid and the key ingredient in aspirin.

Inflammation and the formation of cancer as a result is not a new idea and has been considered for centuries and particularly when in the year 1863 WBCs were found present in high numbers in cancerous tissue by Dr Rudolph Virchow, a German medic and biologist. A vast number of cancers especially those involving epithelial cells have been extremely closely linked to the inflammatory process involving WBCs and associated chemical triggers known as cytokines. It is apparent that the inflammatory process has lost control and instead of protecting tissue by its action can in fact cause tissue to turn cancerous. The process will be explained in some detail below to aid understanding why managing chronic inflammation is so important in the fight against cancer.

Inflammation is your body's response to attack and is an important part of our immune system.

The "attack" can be a large physical attack like a cut, sprained ankle or parasitic worm or much smaller like a bacteria, virus or even an allergen like pollen for example. Inflammation as a part of your immune system that is also a key part of your body's healing capacity. Inflammation is a result of fluid retention and swelling and is linked to redness due to increased blood volume and pain. This inflammation process should be a short-lived and acute part of natural healing. Acute inflammation helps isolate ("quarantine") the affected area and also attract the body's defensive yet highly aggressive White Blood Cells. "Healthy" acute inflammation is short lived and ideally lasts only a matter of days. Acute inflammation is a normal process that protects and heals the body following physical injury or infection. However, if the agent causing the inflammation persists for a prolonged period of time, the inflammation becomes chronic. Chronic inflammation can result from a specific continued attack at the site or from the constant production of these chemical triggers (cytokines) by WBCs. viral or microbial infection, environmental antigen (e.g., pollen), autoimmune reaction, or persistent activation of inflammatory molecules.

The link between inflammation and cancer is significant such that cancers have been linked back to the original cause of the specific acute inflammation event. There are cancers caused as consequence of extended or chronic inflammation at a specific site to an "attack". A few example of these include ulcers within the gut caused by bacteria can lead to gastric cancer, the liver fluke parasite can lead to cancer of the bile ducts coming from the liver and the inflammatory response to the human papilloma virus can lead to genital cancer. Inflammation is a highly complex flow of chemical reactions and cell activities that work together to ideally protect the body. Unfortunately like a lot of highly complex systems in life it is prone to go wrong.

ACUTE INFLAMMATION

During the early stages of acute inflammation trigger chemicals such as prostaglandins and histamine are released by cells to help stimulate the inflammatory response. Acute inflammation following attack starts by first contracting the large supply blood vessels to slow blood flow to the affected area's smaller capillaries, which in turn vasodilate to further slow blood flow. This not only helps isolate the area with increased plasma retention in the tissue but also slows the passage of White Blood Cells which then allows them more time and therefore more chance to stick (adhere) to the capillary endothelial walls. This is essential if they are to squeeze through the walls and get to work in the affected tissue. To help the WBCs do this the endothelial cells of the capillary walls contract and therefore create gaps in the wall for the WBCs to escape into the surrounding tissue. In simple terms the large blood vessels shrink to slow blood flow and the small blood vessels expand and become leaky to allow the WBCs to pass through. These two events lead to the swelling and redness in appearance of the inflamed area. To further help the WBCs get to the affected tissue the endothelial cells of the capillary walls locally become sticky by using InterCellular Adhesion Molecules (ICAMs) which help the WBCs with their own complimentary ICAMs to stick to the capillary wall and squeeze through the gaps. Once WBCs have "escaped" from the blood vessels they help fight the attack and deal with any potential infection. The first WBCs at the site of attack are called neutrophils which attempt to eat and kill any invaders such as bacteria. They do this by using powerful oxidative chemicals (ROS) and antimicrobial proteins such as defensins. As stated earlier these ROS have the capacity to do damage not just to the invader but also surrounding healthy body cells. The neutrophils also release additional chemical triggers such as interleukin (IL)-1, IL-6, prostaglandins and tumor necrosis factor (TNF) which result in further inflammatory action. This WBC "escape" process is known and referred to as extravasation if you do any further reading on this area. Extravasation is controlled by the body's regulating and signalling chemicals known as cytokines (such as Interleukin-1 (IL-1), Interleukin-8 (IL-8), and Tumor Necrosis Factor (TNF). There are many benefits related to acute inflammation the main ones being related to your body marshalling its defence against an attack such that WBCs are concentrated in the right place to be most effective and enabling the start of the healing process. Unfortunately problems can arise if the acute inflammation carries on and moves into chronic inflammation which by its nature lasts much longer from weeks to months to years.

CHRONIC INFLAMMATION
Chronic inflammation can arise from constant acute inflammation or as a consequence of a general malfunction of the immune system. This is exceptionally bad for your body as many of the powerful chemical triggers and markers (such as WBCs, C-Reactive Protein (CRP), Interleukin-1 (IL-1), IL-6, IL-18, TNF, intercellular adhesion molecule-1 (ICAM-1) and vascular cell adhesion molecule-1 (VCAM-1)) related to inflammation build up in concentration and spread throughout the body causing inflammation impacts elsewhere with the body. In essence the inflammation process starts to act on your whole body system instead of a small local area, such that this is referred to as chronic whole body inflammation or systemic inflammation or more commonly just chronic inflammation. The concentration of the chemical triggers and markers mentioned earlier are widely used by researchers and clinicians to verify the degree of inflammation present and the effect on inflammation of different treatments and dietary regimes.

Chronic Inflammation also leads to excessive production and decreased management of Reactive Oxygen Species. As previously stated in the oxidative stress chapters many ROS and their toxic byproducts are themselves heavily linked with cancer growth (i.e. carcinogenic) through their reactions with DNA, their ability to reduce natural cell death (apoptosis), their ability to interfere with natural cell repair and their ability to aid the provision of a new blood supply (angiogenesis) to growing cancer cells.

Chronic Inflammation leads to excessive production of the enzyme called cyclooxygenase-2 (COX-2) which is highly active and unfortunately carcinogenic. COX-2 production is stimulated by cytokines and in particular the chemical triggers IL-1 and TNF. This chronic inflammation is maintained by WBCs which are responsible for the production and release of high levels of Tumour Necrosis Factor (TNF). WBCs (monocytes and macrophages) are active in maintaining chronic inflammation. This excessive and chronic WBCs' activity has been shown to be extremely negative and is accepted to help cancers grow. This is not that surprising when you consider that TNF released by WBCs activates the gene switch chemical Nuclear Factor- kappa B (NFkB). NFkB can then enters the nucleus of a potential tumour cell and turns on production of proteins that stop apoptosis and promote cell proliferation and inflammation.

COX-2 is found in high concentrations within tumours and this enzyme is also believed to help cancerous cells by inhibiting apoptosis and promoting angiogenesis. COX-2 is particularly active in epithelial cancers and especially those of the digestive tract. It is in large part the interaction of both (ROS and COX-2) these carcinogens and TNF in different pathways which leads to the stimulation of NFkB (nuclear factor kappa-light-chain-enhancer of activated B cells).

NFkB plays a lead role in the inflammatory and immune response. NFkB is a common trigger chemical (transcription factor) within the body involved in the regulation of many cell events such as apoptosis and the production of cell adhesion molecules. NFkB is a major chemical trigger which is often called a gene switch due to its ability to turn certain inactive genes on. This linked with TNFs ability to also trigger the development of new blood vessels (angiogenesis) which will then be able to feed the greedy growing cancer with nutrients is a dangerous mixture. As levels of NFkB increase it enters the nucleus of a tumour cell and turns on production of proteins that in turn stop cell death and promote cell differentiation, proliferation and inflammation. There is a clear body of evidence which has shown that activated NFkB is directly linked to inflammation and cancer. NFkB has been found to be excessively high in concentration in several cancers especially during cancer growth and other inflammatory diseases. NFkB clearly enables more rapid tumour growth. Many studies have looked at reducing NFkB levels to try to help in the fight against cancer. It is also important to be aware that NFkB plays an important part in normal cell function but during cancer it is highly active. It has been found to be excessively high in concentration in several cancers especially during cancer growth and other inflammatory diseases.

Just because someone suffers with chronic inflammation it does not mean they are definitely going to get cancer but the chances are higher of this occurring. Equally it is important to acknowledge that NFkBs are also essential for normal healthy cellular function. Over production of NFkB is commonly started as part of the inflammatory response to "attack" and is often activated by TNF. Anything that can inhibit the over-production of NFkB is considered by many researchers and clinicians as highly useful in the fight against cancer, whether that fight is preventative or curative. Many plants contain highly useful chemicals in the fight against cancer which is why **many nutritionists and doctors recommend a diet with a high intake of fruit, nuts and vegetables and why even the UK government is recommending "five – a – day" as part of an attempt to increase the health of the nation.** However there is a lot of food to choose from and we want to focus on those that are most effective in the fight against cancer. There have been many thousands of studies clarifying the health benefits of a "Mediterranean diet" or any diet high in vegetable matter, fibre, low in red meat and regular fish intake etc. There has however been only limited success in specific single food-based research which proves significant health benefits especially in the fight against cancer. It is widely accepted that the human body probably uses the health benefits of a range of food in a complex and an additive manner. I have throughout this book tried to focus on highly researched and evidence-based areas that have the potential to help significantly in the fight against cancer. For this chapter a large focus is placed on those foodstuffs and chemicals which can impact on NFkB production. Of the foodstuffs it appears that **Walnuts and Cloves** in particular have a significant reduction impact on NFkB production both in the degree of impact and speed of action. Not only is this noted in test-tube research but also animal studies. It not only appears that they reduce NFkB production but also that they work well together by reducing inflammation, cell migration and tumour growth. Walnuts are high in antioxidants and Alpha-Linolenic Acid more commonly known as "an Omega 3" fatty acid / oil which is widely regarded as highly beneficial in reducing cholesterol, inflammation and maintaining arterial springiness. Cloves have a long history as plant with extremely powerful medicinal benefits. It is most commonly used to reduce inflammation and pain in the mouth and throat. Cloves are so powerful that they can reduce the pain and inflammation caused by a mouth abscess within an hour of application. It is a powerful taste and is used only sparingly in cooking. Cloves have the ability to kill parasitic worms within the digestive system and antiviral properties and often used as part of a detox. I personally do not recommend more than five of them ground up per day as you may find your gut reacts to them in an undesirable way. Some people enjoy using it as a regular daily herb in their cooking whilst others use 5 of them to make a daily tea drink with them. It has been noted that coffee, oregano and thyme also impact on the production of NFkB to a degree and for most people a nice strong coffee is probably more preferable to a clove tea but it is less likely to be as effective in helping you in the fight against cancer. All inflammatory chemicals have an effect on cells in a range of ways including stimulating angiogenesis, stimulating cell production, inhibiting apoptosis and increasing production of cell adhesion molecules. All of these individually and together can help cause cancer, can help cancers grow and can help certain cancers spread to other sites (metastasis). Much of traditional medicine has shown by inhibiting some of these inflammatory chemicals cancers growth or spread has been halted significantly.

Chronic inflammation is abnormal and does not benefit the body; in fact, chronic inflammation is involved in a number of disease states. With the natural aging process chronic inflammation is much more common and can have serious long term negative effects on the body that often lead to disease. Very high levels of chronic inflammation chemicals such as IL-6 have been noted in patients with advanced cancers. The oxidative damage linked with chronic inflammation is accepted as a significant factor in the formation of cancer. It is widely accepted by modern medicine that chronic inflammation is in fact one of the main common factors to all chronic degenerative diseases. These diseases are many and varied but all directly or indirectly linked to chronic inflammation. Chronic inflammation has been linked to very many inflammatory ailments, infections and diseases such as asthma, gastritis, Crohn's disease, bowel disease, rheumatoid arthritis, diabetes, atherosclerosis, obesity, heart disease, multiple sclerosis, Alzheimer's disease and very many different cancers.

Chronic inflammation can result in considerable tissue damage due to having leaky capillaries and high WBCs activity for longer periods than is healthy. WBCs are highly active and as stated before highly aggressive. Associated with the WBCs prolonged activity there is a significant increase in concentration of ROS and powerful protein destroying enzymes at the site which can be highly detrimental to cells causing substantial oxidative damage such as cancer. Excessive WBCs activity can lead to severe tissue damage.

ANTIHISTAMINES & INFLAMMATION CONTROL

When there is consistent inflammation (and even some cancers) traditional medical treatment involves the use of anti-inflammatory drugs such as antihistamines or corticosteroids to relieve the symptoms, damage and manage the cancer growth. **Cetirizine** is an over-the-counter antihistamine available in many countries without prescription commonly used to alleviate the symptoms of hay fever and other allergies. It is also used to help combat excessive inflammation such as in cases of hives. It has many properties and interestingly it has also been used to reduce chronic inflammation, immune system malfunction and skin lesions. Although available over the counter it is important to remember that high doses and long term use can result in annoying and serious side-effects such as drying of the mucosal linings in the mouth and nose especially, stomach upset and even blurred vision. Cetirizine can be very helpful in your fight against cancer as it is able to limit the production of key chemicals involved in chronic inflammation. The reduced production of ICAM-1, IL-6 and IL-8 caused by Cetirizine is of significant benefit in reducing the impacts of chronic inflammation. The ability of Cetirizine to also limit the production of NFkB is probably the most important when considering your fight against cancer. Many have found it useful in helping in their fight against cancer by using it to the maximum dose stated on the pack for a period of two weeks. As always seek medical advice before incorporating this and any medicine or supplement into your diet regime. It is less likely to work as effectively for brain cancer as the active chemical only manages to cross the blood brain barrier slightly although this does not stop many people using it.

Antihistamines have a significant impact on cellular histamine and cellular cytochrome P450 enzymes, both of which are linked to cell growth and multiplication. Cetirizine as already mentioned is very useful in the fight against cancer as it also reduces intercellular adhesion molecules and subsequent inflammatory activity. Cetirizine is an antihistamine which is commonly taken without prescription for hay fever.

Ranitidine (Zantac) is used to block acid production in the stomach, for indigestion, acid reflux, heartburn, ulcer treatment and treatment of Zollinger-Ellison syndrome. Ranitidine works by blocking histamine H2 receptors in the gut (similar to Cimetidine known as "Tagamet" in US). Side effects from Ranitidine are unusual but can include diarrhoea, dizziness or rashes which usually do not last. Occasionally slight enlargement of the breasts in men has been reported in Ranitidine users but usually stops when treatment ends.

There has been research published in the respected Cancer Journal which suggests that **Cimetidine** can help survival in some people with colon cancer if Cimetidine is taken several days before surgical intervention. In one particular study patients took 800mg Cimetidine twice daily for five days before the operation with improved results. Cimetidine does stimulate the immune system and this is thought to be part of the cause of the increase in survival rates.

Ranitidine and Cimetidine are antihistamines that are known to interfere with cytochrome P450 enzyme system. Additionally they have shown to have anticancer effects, which include reducing ROS production, interfering with, cancer cell multiplication and angiogenesis. Both have a similar action but Cimetidine appears to be more widely praised. However Cimetidine has been more extensively researched and so the more positive results for its action might be slightly more biased. Cimetidine has been shown to be beneficial for kidney function in patients having chemotherapy involving cisplatin. Cisplatin is a powerful drug which is known to cause kidney damage in large doses. Both these antihistamines are also thought to help in the fight against cancers, but especially colon and gastric cancers by interfering with histamine's ability to promote cell growth.

It has been argued that by controlling the inflammatory response to some degree that cancer prevention is realistically possible in people with a past history or family history of cancer. There are a great number of studies looking at the long term impacts of using **Non-Steroidal Anti-Inflammatory Drugs (NSAIDs)**. In particular several large population studies lasting over decades have indicated that extended NSAIDs use has reduced the relative risk of getting colon cancer by close to 50%. They are many significant studies which have also shown that use of NSAIDs in patients with certain cancers have resulted in substantial shrinkage or regression of tumours.

Non-steroidal anti-inflammatory drugs (NSAIDs) especially **Aspirin** have shown promising results in a range of solid cancers and may have significant cancer prevention capabilities for melanomas following lab tests on melanoma cells. **These lab tests have shown that NSAIDs can induce apoptosis and slow cancer growth and limit the attack on non-cancerous cells by cancer cells.** It is has been noted by researchers and clinicians that lots of cancers have higher levels of COX-2 enzyme and prostaglandins present. For over 40 years it has been known that Aspirin could reduce the production of prostaglandins which are powerful signaling chemicals created by cells. Cells produce significantly higher levels of prostaglandins during times of increased COX-2 concentration especially during inflammation. This link led to further scientific research which reviewed NSAIDs possible treatments or preventative medicines for a wider range of cancers including breast, stomach, pancreas, urinary tract, lung, and prostate. It is accepted that Aspirin and many NSAIDs work in a positive way in the fight against cancer by limiting the production of the bad COX-2 enzyme. Aspirin also does the same unfortunately to the good COX-1 enzyme which leads to the damage of the stomach lining over time. COX enzymes are directly involved in the production of prostaglandins, which are a range of highly potent chemicals produced by cells which act as triggers for other actions for example cell growth, vasodilation and bronchoconstriction. COX-2 enzymes enable production of prostaglandins which are involved in the inflammatory response and tumour growth and hence why COX-2 enzymes when considering the fight against cancer have been called the bad COX enzymes.

COX-2 is normally absent in most cells and tissues but it is produced in large amounts in response to inflammation and its linked chemical reactions. Many recent clinical, longitudinal and large population studies show that long term use of aspirin and NSAIDs can significantly reduce the occurrence of many different cancers such as lymphoma, lung, breast, bladder and colon cancers. In particular it seems that a prostaglandin caused by COX-2 stimulation known as prostaglandin E-2 (PGE-2) causes cancer growth by interfering with chemical reactions which control key cell functions such as cell division, apoptosis, blood supply and movement. However all this positive news about Aspirin's and NSAIDs capabilities should be tempered with the knowledge that very high doses over a long period of time can not only cause mild side effects but also potentially serious damage to the heart and circulatory system. So it is not going to be recommended to take high doses but more widespread use of low doses of Aspirin is occurring for other inflammatory diseases such as arthritis and inflammatory bowel disease.

Aspirin's main method of action appears to be by interfering with the COX-2 production and thus the production of certain prostaglandins. Many researchers have found that there are additional possible anti-cancer properties of Aspirin and other NSAIDs. These include their ability to interact with other signaling systems and sites such as the Par-4 gene and NFkB signaling. It is important to be aware that this is test-tube research with the doses used not possible the human body due to toxic effects. This is not to say that the power of aspirin should be overlooked but care and guidance should be sought regarding its use in your fight against cancer.

Aspirin is likely to some degree prevent colon and other cancers through inhibition of COX-2 and NFkB. It is accepted that COX-2 enzymes encourage excessive inflammation and cell multiplication and that COX-2 is present in high concentrations in colon and other cancers. Positive results have been noted by attempts to control COX-2 levels in various solid cancers by using NSAIDs. Melanoma cells which are some of the most aggressive cancer cells have had their growth reduced and cell death (apoptosis) induced by the use of NSAIDs. Regular aspirin use after the diagnosis of colon cancer is associated with lower risk of colon cancer growth and early mortality. This is especially likely in people with cancers that have high levels of COX-2 enzymes present.

Aspirin and calcium may reduce recurrence of adenomas and incidence of advanced adenomas in individuals with an increased risk of colon cancer. COX-2 inhibitors may decrease polyp number in patients prone to this. There is evidence that aspirin reduces the incidence of colon cancer in the general population.

A lot of research shows that even low levels of aspirin use can reduce the impact and risk of several cancers. In animal tests Aspirin has been shown to reduce the growth of a range of cancers such as cancers of the lung, skin, breast, prostate and colon. For example in a statistical review of a range of human longitudinal studies it was found that there is an approximately 50% reduction in risk for colon cancer with daily low dose aspirin use. Many studies showing other good results have seen that even weekly low dose aspirin use over a long period seem to have an impact. It has also been shown to reduce the re-occurrence of certain already treated cancers as well. There are no definitive answers as always on dosage with regard to Aspirin and colon cancer which will obviously vary person to person anyway. As a rough indicator some human studies indicate that doses above 75mg daily did not result in any further improvement but that daily doses lower than 30mg are less effective but clearly as always this should be discussed with your doctor.

If you are to integrate the use of aspirin in to your fight against cancer it is important to remember that the significant use of aspirin and other NSAIDs is associated with bad side effects such as nausea, dyspepsia, gastritis, abdominal pain, an inflamed and possibly bleeding stomach lining and ulcers. The possible ways aspirin works to inhibit the NFkB is not fully understood but the fact that it does is consistently shown. NFkB is active in many cancers and controls a wide range of genes involved with the inflammatory and immune process as well as cell growth and death.

Azelaic acid is found in **wheat, rye and barley**. It acts as a signaling chemical in plants which induces the buildup of salicylic acid as part of its "immune" system. Salicylic acid is a chemical which is very similar to aspirin. Azelaic acid used to treat acne has been found to have significant anti-cancer properties for a range of cancers including skin cancers. Research in the lab has shown it to have the ability to induce cell death in cancer cells as well as reduce it from spreading by regulating mitochondrial activity in normal cells and interfering with or destroying the mitochondrial activity of cancer cells.

Research in humans has shown that Azelaic acid reduces melanoma tumour size and spread. Azelaic acid is very flexible in that it can be applied to the skin or given orally and intravenously. Unlike many other treatments for cancer it does not seem to have any significant toxic effects even with large doses. There is obviously a lot more research necessary but Azelaic acid would appear to be a very powerful and focused chemical which could be very useful in your fight against cancer.

Aspirin and Low Density Lipids (LDLs) which carry cholesterol

LDLs can transport cholesterol into the arterial walls and attract WBCs that then form into plaques which are commonly increased in atherosclerosis and heart disease leading to the increased risk of heart attack and strokes. Remember also excessive activity of WBCs causing oxidative stress and chronic inflammation impacts. This is why LDLs containing cholesterol are often referred to as "bad" cholesterol. When LDLs are oxidized they can cause even more risk of plaques and damage.

The oxidation of LDL occurs when the LDL particles react with ROS among other things. The oxidized LDL then becomes more reactive with the cells around it, which can then produce significant tissue damage. Some of the things that appear to increase levels of oxidized LDL unsurprisingly include consuming a diet that is high in fats especially trans-fat, a poor metabolism, smoking and diabetes.

Once LDLs become oxidized, they concentrate in the arteries' endothelial lining including main arteries such as the, carotid, aorta and coronary artery. Once there, it encourages the accumulation of WBCs. This interaction leads not only to the growth of potentially dangerous plaques but also oxidative stress and chronic inflammation. These by themselves as already discussed can lead to a range of diseases including atherosclerosis, heart disease, stroke and cancer.

Oxidative stress and oxidized-Low Density Lipids (ox-LDL) both alter endothelial biochemistry by activating an ox-LDL receptor site called Lectin-type OXidized LDL receptor-1 or LOX-1 for short. This LOX-1 activation has been shown to lead to further oxidative stress in endothelial cells and significant chronic inflammation. Many studies have proved that ox-LDLs cause significant oxidative stress within cells and thereby can activate NFkB and a dangerous inflammatory state within cells.

Vitamin E is highly protective and consists of well-known fat soluble antioxidants has been studied in detail for their impact on ox-LDLs. Well respected studies have shown that Vitamin E (both alpha and gamma tocopherol) help stop ox-LDLs interacting with the LOX-1 sites and make it more difficult for WBCs to stick to arterial walls. It is believed that combining Vitamin E with aspirin use can limit the problems caused by ox-LDLs to a large degree. Vitamin E is highly protective as it also helps manage the damage to the heart and the cancer risk of such drugs as Adriamycin, daunomycin, dimethylhydrazine as well as ROS.

Dipyridamole, like aspirin, inhibits platelet adhesion, and thus tends to prevent the vascular thrombosis of heart attacks and strokes. The European Stroke Prevention Study was a large 2 year trial looking at the use of 300 mg of dipyridamole a day with aspirin. They found fantastic results for decreasing stroke deaths by 50%, but also they reduced cancer related deaths by 25%. It is believed by many that the reduction in cancer-related deaths is because dipyridamole has an anti-inflammatory action by reducing the formation of inflammatory cytokines. It also helps to stop the action of the Mengovirus. Mengovirus if not stopped interacts with cell RNA and is able to reduce the body's immune response. Dipyridamole is widely prescribed by oncologists for a range of long term cancer patients. It is a medication that can be obtained in many countries without a prescription via the internet but of course must be used only following consultation with your doctor. Based on its positive action counteracting an RNA virus it would make sense for a scientific review of this chemical and colchicine in the fight against the Wuhan Virus of 2019 commonly known as Corona virus or CoVID-19.

In conclusion it is widely accepted by most researchers and clinicians that chronic inflammation leads to an associated increased and hard to manage WBC activity. With this constant high level of WBC activity there is an increased concentration of longer duration of ROS and cytokines, which could possibly be directly linked to tumour stimulation and formation.

Clearly chronic inflammation is far from an ideal body response in people with cancer already as it can encourage cancer tumours to grow. It is therefore not such a bad idea to think of anti-inflammatory solutions to help you in your fight against cancer. It is highly likely that this is already part of your medication if on a chemotherapy treatment and so as always make sure your consult your physician before taking any steps down this road and before following the "Jobs to do".

Jobs to Do

1. Consider taking low dose aspirin, calcium, and cetirizine

2. Ask doctor about **dipyridamole**

3. Eat more walnuts cloves, oregano thyme and coffee

4. Consider taking Ranitidine/Cimetidine 1000mg/day for 2 weeks with review

5. Increase Vitamin E and eat natural Yoghurt with ground flax seeds

6. Eat low cholesterol diet in particular no trans fat

7. Ask doctor about considering Azelaic Acid with Aspirin especially in melanoma cases

AS PREVIOUSLY STATED NUMEROUS TIMES THIS IS A PERSONAL CHOICE WHICH SHOULD BE MADE IN CONSULTATION WITH YOUR DOCTOR.

Chapter 10: Placebo Effect

The placebo effect is a widely heard of but poorly understood phenomenon whereby a patient's illness or complaint can be improved by an otherwise scientifically invalidated treatment. This is widely thought to occur because the patients think that the treatment will work. A good example is when a mother kisses a scraped knee better. Following many scraped knees etc. and reinforcement of this process a belief structure in children and also adults is instilled, that a comforting feeling of improvement follows a "kiss it better" treatment. The same can be said for the belief that doctors make you better.... It is also true that an illness or complaint can be improved with a regular medicine with an added bonus of placebo effect.

The placebo effect can be a physiological response brought on by the power of the mind or a purely psychological response to treatment. The physiological response brought on by a psychological response can be beneficial and even a purely psychological response or belief helps many patients deal better with their ailment. Any positive response is better from a patient's point of view than a negative one. The problem that modern medicine and science has with the placebo effect is that it cannot understand it fully, bottle it up and sell it on. The placebo effect can be used by both traditional medicine and complementary medicine to prove or disprove their points of view, when really for the sake of the individual patient in front of them they should try to harness it as a power to help healing.

Generally it is agreed that all medicines and treatments can induce the placebo effect, but only those that have a healing effect above this changeable percentage produced by a placebo that are classified as truly worthwhile or significantly curative. Why if the numbers are big enough does the placebo effect percentage change? There are a multitude of theories trying to answer this apart from the obvious differences in social beliefs and differences in severity of illnesses.

The exact numbers vary according to researcher and pathology but generally a placebo seems to work 20% of the time. Even if it is considerably less than this number for cancer it still has the potential to be a powerful ally in the fight against cancer. The strange thing about the placebo effect is that many people believe that only highly suggestible and stupid people can possibly benefit from the placebo effect. Many studies have disproved this theory and in fact the placebo effect is a lot more complex than this in its action.

Trying to harness the placebo effect is probably a useful exercise for cancer fighters as it may improve your survival chances significantly if you are one of the people who is lucky enough to be affected by the placebo effect.

It is believed that the placebo effect is highly reliant on the patient's past experiences and belief structure such that it could be a socially conditioned response that some people are more susceptible to. For example there are those people who just by going to the doctor feel better because they have memories of feeling better in the past having been to the doctor or taken a particular medicine. The brain is a very powerful and little understood organ which has been seen to produce and release endorphins of higher levels in some people following a visit to the doctors or taking a medicine. These endorphins are chemicals which act on our bodies like painkillers and give a feeling of well-being. There have been studies on doctors' bedside manner which have seen improvements in their positivity relating to lower stress levels and stress hormones in patients. Stress hormones are very powerful and complex hormones which interact with the endocrine system and metabolic processes. Constant and high levels of stress hormones are known to have significant effects which impact on a range of illnesses and systems. High levels of cortisol for example are known to affect the body's immune system by inhibiting and interfering with the inflammatory response in particular the normal functioning of T-lymphocytes.

The positive outlook of the doctor combined with the patient's faith in the treatment may also lead to a lessening of stress and anxiety in the patient. Stress and anxiety adversely affect the body and increase patients' focus on symptoms. Reduction of stress and anxiety may subsequently reduce some physical symptoms, as a secondary effect that is exacerbated by stress and anxiety.

In many studies it has been seen that larger placebo pills are more effective than smaller ones, as are coloured ones over white pills. This would tend to indicate it is not just the receiving of a supposed treatment but also the person's belief that bigger is more powerful and that a deep mental relationship with colour causes a belief that something with colour is more powerful than something white. It has been shown that red placebo pills can "act" more effectively as stimulants whereas "green" placebo pills can "act" as anti-depressants. In history there have been cases of pseudo operations where the patient has been anaesthetized and had the "theatre" of the operating theatre with accompanying surgeon but nothing actually done and the patient has noted improvement.

It is interesting to note that doctors researching the placebo effect have noticed that large dummy (placebo) pills are more effective than small ones, and coloured ones are more effective than white; showing that the expectation of the strength of the pill affects patients' responses. Studies related to branding have shown that well known branded packaging and generic packaging used for exactly the same drug have shown interesting results. It has been demonstrated that branding clearly does work better at a placebo medical level. There are cultural differences between specific beliefs, but the most useful and fascinating fact is that placebo effects occur with all cultures and are not absolutely reliant on being directly believed as a treatment, although the more belief the better. It does show that on a both a mental and a physiological basis that humans can be directly influenced by placebo treatments. There obviously is a big difference between feeling better which some placebo treatment induce and actually recovering which other placebo treatments induce. When considered it can be seen that all forms of treatment can exhibit the placebo phenomenon. The power of the human brain and how it interacts with the endocrine system is not fully understood, but it should not be underestimated. This may explain why often people with deep spiritual beliefs or meditation can overcome seemingly extremely poor prognoses and maybe why religious employees such as priests have higher life expectancies than most or it may be that their lives are less stressful and dangerous in general terms.

Although there is the widespread belief that placebo effects are theoretically possible for any pathology and any treatment there are few extensive and detailed studies. Many researchers agree that placebos appear to have most impact in pain management and autonomic nervous system disorders. The autonomic nervous system is a highly complex and integrated system that exerts wide acting control on a range of physiological processes for a wide range of tissues and organs. The placebo effect is often referred to as a psycho-physiological effect. It is therefore not beyond belief that better control of this system could be of benefit to cancer fighters.

The problem of harnessing the placebo effect in the fight against cancer is far from easy. The power of the active mind to impact on human physiology has been shown to be not fully understood. However it is known that by meditation and breathing techniques that both pulse and blood pressure can be reduced along with improved Oxygen and Carbon Dioxide exchange. Also that meditation helps people alleviate anxiety and arrive at a state of mental relaxation. Apart from anxiety leading to the increased production of stress hormones it is known that anxiety activates the hypothalamus and pituitary areas of the brain leading to the potential for further impacts on the endocrine system. The majority of current cancer research is now focusing on endocrinology as a route to greater understanding of non-environmental/internal causes of cancer. Endorphins are often referred to as the "happy hormones" (neurotransmitters) that are released by the pituitary gland and hypothalamus during and following exercise and other thoughts, feelings or activities (such as love, excitement, eating spicy food, orgasm.

How endorphins interact with brain receptor sites is not fully understood but it is known that they give a sense of wellbeing. A sense of wellbeing is often a body sign of improved health and vitality and maybe a useful remnant of physical evolution which helps keep us physically fit and aid survival of the species. It might be that the placebo effect is also in fact an evolutionary remnant design to help the species help itself survive. In simple terms a cancer fighter who feels better is probably likely to be a better fighter both physically and mentally than one that does not.

Epidemiological, laboratory and clinical studies have shown clear links between infection with its associated inflammation and many cancers. Natural Killer cells are often stimulated into action following an infection. These Natural Killer cells are White Blood Cells known as lymphocytes which are a critical part of the immune system. Natural Killer (NK) cells recognize cancer cells and mutant cells infected with viruses and then attack them. NK cells' ability to attack cancer cells is controlled by multiple mechanisms such as direct cytotoxic activity against target cells. As a consequence many studies are reviewing how to effectively use or stimulate NK Cells to help in the fight against cancer in activating NK cells physiological functions and reducing the body's own inflammatory response.

High levels of chronic stress are well known to increase cancer growth, which is why there has been an increase in stress reduction techniques such as meditation in complementary cancer care. These non-drug stress reduction techniques have been shown to help the immunity and to reduce tumor growth of patients with cancer. The power of the brain and its impact on cancer will be further examined in the next chapter on laughter and positivity generally.

Jobs to Do

There are lots of ways you can use the information in this chapter most of them are linked to thinking yourself well but also from de-stressing and meditating more to reviewing your religious beliefs.

1. Colour your pills with red food dye.

2. Take big supplement tablets from well-known brands.

3. Really listen to your doctor and or health practitioner and believe that they will help you.
4. Attend Relaxation / Meditation / Tai Chi classes.

5. Do some regular vigorous exercise if able which helps release endorphins, remember vigorous exercise can include sex which also helps release endorphins!

6. Eat some of your favourite meals including dark chocolate.

7. Positively visualise your body's natural killer cells killing specifically your cancer.

Chapter 11: Laughter – Is the best doctor a comedian?

Chronic stress may contribute to immune system deficits and has been linked to chronic inflammation. Cortisone is immunosuppressant (by dampening tumour surveillance cells and by making natural killer cells less effective) and adrenalin kills lymphocytes. Addressing stress, in general, may go some way to reducing the risk of cancer. Measuring chronic stress is replete with difficulties; we don't know how long, or at what age, or whether there are relevant potentiating/mitigating factors that might be part of the final analysis in understanding the role of stress in the development of cancer.

It is widely accepted by both scientists and the general public alike that high levels of stress and anxiety cause significant physiological changes to your body. Many of these physiological changes include the increased release of powerful stress hormones such as adrenocorticotropic hormone (ACTH), epinephrine (adrenaline), norepinephrine (nor-adrenaline) and cortisol. Stress hormones are known to impact the metabolic system at a cellular level. If stress hormones are maintained at too high a level for too long a period there can be serious weakening of the immune system and the natural balance of Sodium and Potassium ions can be significantly altered. Not only are these classic powerful stress hormones released due to high levels of stress, but whole body effects are noted due to the influence that stress can have on a wide range of other hormones and chemical signalers such as thyroid hormone, growth hormone, insulin, glucagon, prolactin, gonadotrophin, neurohormones and cytokines. Laughter is a natural way that you can help to reduce stress as well as enjoy improving your health status.

It is not a new idea that both physical and psychological stress can have a detrimental effect on health. In fact right at the beginnings of western medicine in Greece the doctors of the time were concerned with people's psychological type and the link with their temperamental or constitutional type. In fact the term humour which can describe your happiness level or likelihood of laughing is in fact derived from the ancient Greek medical usage of the word. The types are known as the four humours of Hippocrates and were key to using the medicine of the time. It can be seen from these four humours names; sanguine, choleric, melancholic and phlegmatic, that they are descriptions that relate to a person's temperament (extrovert and sociable, ambitious and impulsive, introverted and sensitive, reserved and relaxed, respectively). Although in ancient Greek times there were no random placebo-controlled trials of medicines such as today's requirement for scientific observation and theory, it was a time when the subject of mathematics was treated with reverence. In relation to our discussion about laughter the renowned physician Galen (much of whose work was significantly ahead of its time and is still held with high regard) interestingly noted that the melancholic (unhappy) person was most likely to present with cancer. There are of course many modern day anecdotal examples of people suffering great illness after a highly stressful event either physical or mental in nature. Much research has shown that stress exerts a significant impact on a range of important physiological systems such as the endocrine, lymphatic, immune and sympathetic nervous systems. These significant impacts can in certain susceptible individuals lead to the occurrence of significant illnesses and diseases.

How the brain exactly reacts to laughter at a hormonal and physiological level is poorly understood. It appears that initially something visual or aural causes neuro-stimulation of the anterior supplementary motor area leading to physical laughter. This highly specialized area appears to focus on speech and fine motor skills and it appears unclear the purpose of laughter at a physiological level but clearly it is an important part of a social animal's expression and acceptance by the group. Just as speech/communication and group grooming is important for primates' social behaviour. Obviously an improved immune system is a necessary requirement for a social animal to reduce the chances of picking up species-specific diseases. This whole area raises more questions and theories than it answers, but regardless the cancer fighter can use this knowledge to help plan a health strategy.

The human purpose of laughter is far from clear, but it does appear to be a universal and fundamental if not primitive reaction or response that the human body derives some increased survival benefit. In fact this survival benefit to the species and its linked social function was considered in some depth by Charles Darwin. If we consider that your average six week old baby will smile and not much later will giggle when their mother plays peek-a-boo with them. This laughter it can be assumed is an essential part of bonding for the new arrival to the family and allows for greater acceptance and integration of new mouth to feed! Like mutual grooming for other primates it seems laughter aids social cohesion of a group and a feeling of understanding and security. This tends to explain the likelihood of increased laughing at a joke when in the company of others so-called infectious laughter. This social company effect is well understood by the makers of TV comedy shows hence the use of "canned laughter" to help their programme's laugh per minute ratio. The social and cultural context of laughter of a particular group leads to increased cohesion of the group. This is sometimes demonstrated by immigrants who find it difficult to laugh at another cultural group's jokes and miss this shared humour aspect of their past lives the most. Laughter and its reduction in stress hormones etc. seems to be closely related but almost opposite to the primitive "fight or flight" response which humans have if stimulated by a potentially dangerous stimulus e.g. the roar of a tiger. Stress hormones are essential if you under threat to make you able to act but if the danger passes then these stress hormone levels need to be normalised and is possible that laughter achieves this need. Physiologically laughter is similar to tears in that it "enables" this normalisation process to occur and gives a release from this state of tension. This is one reason why many people feel physically better for a good laugh or a good cry. It is also why some people can end up crying after or during a good laugh. From a neurophysiological point of view laughter is highly complex and involves many areas of specific brain activity. It can be thought of as almost whole brain activity as many believe that the cognitive areas of the frontal lobe aid the understanding of the joke or stimulus, the motor control areas trigger the many physical movements caused by laughter and that the emotional areas are the main centres of activity.

Laughter is a physical activity which helps the lymphatic system move lymph more effectively which helps the body's immune system function more effectively. Really good hearty laughter also helps improve the oxygenation of blood by the increased frequency and depth of breathing. The increased levels of oxygen helps cells' mitochondria metabolise glucose more effectively and thereby reduce the production of dangerous toxins that occur during anaerobic respiration. During laughter it has been noted that your pulse quickens and so your body also gets a boost to its circulation thus also further improving oxygenation of cells. Those of you that remember being in fits of laughter know that the body can't maintain this for too long as it is physically exhausting. However a regular laugh does seem to be good for you physically as well as mentally. The mental wellbeing following laughter is as a result of a range of chemicals in your body being released or activated. Many of these chemicals don't just help you feel better and relieve depression but also improve your health. Chemicals such as interleukins, endorphins and serotonin help your body in a range of anti-inflammatory and immune system boosting ways.

Using laughter as medicine is far from a new idea. In the 14th century the benefit of laughter in healthcare was recognised. The famous French surgeon Henri de Mondeville is known to have used laughter to aid recovery from serious surgery. He wrote that it was the doctor's duty to try and ensure the patient's life was full of happiness which included "allowing his relatives and special friends to cheer him and by having someone tell him jokes." In the USA there has long been acceptance that happiness and laughter has a useful medical function. Before the Second World War in America polio was epidemic and on many of the children's polio wards they funded clowns to entertain the children with an emphasis on laughter. There is the world famous case of Dr. Norman Cousins who in 1960s was diagnosed with a potentially fatal illness and used laughter in an extreme way. Rather than trusting the unguaranteed treatments recommended by the specialist doctors he discharged himself from hospital and went to a hotel. There he proceeded to watch all his favourite comedy films and TV programmes, which included Charlie Chaplin and Marx Brothers films amongst others. He believes that he laughed so long and so much that it had a physiological effect that cured him. Not that I am recommending such an extreme approach but clearly it is useful to integrate and use this knowledge in your own fight against cancer. If you are interested in his story then he wrote a book about his journey called "Anatomy of an Illness."

The sayings "Stop! I can't breathe" and "I nearly died laughing" are often used to describe how hard you were laughing but like most sayings there is often some truth linked to them. It is extremely rare but it is possible due to asthma attack, heart attack or laughter-induced syncope that laughter could lead to death. When laughter-induced syncope presents in a person it is commonly found in families and is therefore believed to be genetic in nature. In theory the laughter-caused heart attack could happen to anyone with a weak heart, however again this seems to be exceptionally rare and is more likely a rare inherited heart rhythm abnormality. It is believed that the famous death by laughter in the UK of a man who had a heart attack whilst watching "The Goodies" (a comedy TV series in the 1970s) in fact had this rare heart abnormality. This rather morbid information should not scare you too much as death by laughter is extremely rare, however you should see that it demonstrates that laughter is a very powerful whole body physiological stimulator. Conversely and interestingly this is an area which has generated interest in the field of preventive cardiology, as it is becomes clear that laughter stimulation could be useful in the prevention of heart disease. The theories are linked to a reduction in stress which appears linked to fat and cholesterol deposits in the coronary arteries.

There is highly repeatable scientific research which shows that laughter is highly beneficial to our health and well-being but because it seems too simplistic its medical benefits are often overlooked by traditional medicine. It is understandable that traditional medicine might find it difficult to prescribe laughter to be taken in regular doses but the phrase laughter is the best medicine does come to mind! The proven health benefits include improved oxygenation and respiration. Lowering stress hormones, improving immune function, lowering blood pressure whilst improving cardiac and vascular function improving muscle function and improving pain management and enhancing our "feel good factor" by the release of endorphins.

It is accepted that cancers can occur or grow faster due to inflammatory processes. Recent research studies in the fields of neuro-immunomodulation and neuropharmacology have shown that during severe depression there are pro-inflammatory responses or effects that occur involving cytokines. In many cases it has been shown that some antidepressants also have an impact on the immune system. The body creates its own natural "antidepressants" such as serotonin and these are encouraged to be released by laughter and physical activity. Studies reviewing serotonin levels have noted that increased levels often lead to important anti-inflammatory responses or effects involving Interleukin 6 & 10 (IL-6 & IL-10), Interferon-gamma, T Helper Lymphocyte Cells and importantly Tumour Necrosis Factor (TNF).

A happy disposition or positive mental attitude is considered one of the key elements of good health. This idea is not new but has been reflected on by philosophers and physicians since Plato and Hippocrates. Apart from common sense, this concept has been verified by more recent research such that regular thoughts and emotions seem to play a key part in determining the length and quality of life. Research has shown that pessimistic individuals have poorer health, are prone to depression, are more frequent users of medical and mental health care delivery systems and show more cognitive decline and impaired immune function as they get older. Also it appears to be consistently shown that pessimists and have a shorter survival rate compared to optimists.

The importance of mental positivity to health in general and the immune system specifically has been regularly researched and the links have led to the creation of a relatively new scientific field, psychoneuroimmunology. This area proves that the belief of the links between mind and body are no longer just the preserve of "New Age hippies" and in fact that the hippies were way ahead of traditional science. Research is showing repeatedly that somehow every part of the immune system is linked to the brain and its function, whether by direct nervous transmission or through a complex interdependent system of chemical messengers and hormones. It is being shown that every brain thought, emotion, and experience sends a message to the immune system which either helps or impairs its function. In simple terms it is being repeatedly proved that positivity, like joy, happiness, and optimism enhances immune system function, but negativity, like depression, sadness, and pessimism impairs immune system function. Research shows that optimistic people have better ratios of helper to suppressor T-cells than those of pessimistic people. This leads to optimists having increased secretory immunoglobulin-A function, natural killer cell activity, and cell-mediated immunity.

The immune system is of great importance in not only preventing cancer but also fighting it. It has been shown to have negativity along with other factors has a measurable impact. For example one study showed that smokers who are suffering from depression have a significantly greater risk of cancer than smokers who are not.

A lot of research has been on the effect on natural killer cells of depression and negativity. There is repeatable evidence that depression and negativity reduces either the number or functional ability of natural killer cells. The study of personality types and cancer has shown that although not universal or categorically causal there is a link between reduced natural killer cell activity and people who suppress anger, avoid conflict, and have a feeling of helplessness with an extreme response to stress.

There is also a negative effect on a cell's ability to repair damage to DNA linked to negativity and depression. As we know the majority of cancer-causing chemicals achieve this by causing damage to the cell's DNA. A crucial process in the cell's fight against cancer is the enzyme action in the cell's nucleus responsible for the repair or disposal of damaged DNA. Repeatable research has shown that negativity and stress alter these DNA repair processes. A recent study proved that lymphocytes from depressed patients had a reduced capability to repair DNA damaged by x-ray radiation.

Not only does negativity have a negative impact on the immune system's function but also research in psychoneuroimmunology has shown that positivity can have a positive impact on the immune system's function. Once again the similarities between cardiovascular health and the immune system are noted in how they respond to negativity and positivity of mental attitude. It has been noted that incidence of coronary heart disease (with occurrences of high blood pressure, heart attack and angina) in older men over a longitudinal study was greater in pessimistic men than optimistic men. Highly optimistic men had a 45% lower risk for angina pectoris, heart attack, and heart disease death than men reporting high levels of pessimism.

With all this knowledge it makes sense health wise to work towards being more optimistic. In fact there are studies reviewing if you can learn optimism or change a pessimistic into an optimist by use of psychological techniques, such as cognitive therapy and positive interventions. Just like in the majority of self-help books it is important not just what happens to your body but how you deal with it. It appears just like getting your body healthy by training it also appears you can get your personal outlook improved by training. Training your outlook to be positive and optimistic requires regular practice and mental conditioning. This can be achieved changing the voice in your head to be more positive and conditioning it to be optimistic and reminding yourself to banish negative thoughts. This can be achieved by seeing a setback as a chance to learn by asking what can I learn from this bad experience so that there is some good that will come from it. Regularly expressing genuine gratitude for people and things to people also helps grow optimism. Many people have found benefit by reviewing and asking themselves what they are most proud of in their lives and what makes them most happy now.

Also by setting positive and achievable goals using positive language it has been shown to improve optimism and definitely not calling it a "bucket" list. It is important to define the goal in positive terms and in the present tense. If of course you are severely depressed it is better to seek help via professional counselling or cognitive therapy as these will likely yield more effective results quicker.

The benefits to the immune system of laughter have been shown many times in ill people. There are studies which show improved immune function in diabetic patients following exposure to laughter-inducing videos. There are studies which show improved blood circulation due to the increased vaso-dilation of the endothelial tissue of blood vessels following exposure to laughter-inducing videos. The list of repeatable research is from highly recognised and independent clinical researchers from around the world. Many studies have shown the physiological and biochemical benefits of laughter but interestingly studies also show that even anticipating laughter can improve our blood biochemistry. It has been shown that by being told that you are about to watch a funny film actually decreases the levels of stress hormones such as cortisol and adrenaline found in blood. This makes sense if we think about the other side of the coin when stress hormones are used by the body in preparation for the so called "fight or flight" response following a body threat where negative anticipation leads to an increase in these hormones to make the body more able to respond to the threat. The benefits to blood biochemistry of laughter and the anticipation of laughter have been shown to last up to 24 hours for some people. So downloading, renting or buying your favourite funny films DVDs, videos and looking forward to them is likely to be highly useful in your fight against cancer and at the very least will make you feel better!

Jobs to do

Laughter is a great weapon in the fight against cancer as it is not painful usually and enjoyable to implement into your health strategy. Other important health therapies such as relaxation, exercise or diet regimes require a major commitment and are often hard to regularly incorporate into your daily routine when compared to having a giggle.

- Watch comedies in the form of funny movies and TV programmes or even go and see a comedian perform live. It is important to vary the type of comedy stimulus as otherwise it is less likely to make us laugh. Try watching some old classics like Laurel and Hardy for a change.
- Spend time with fun friends that make you smile and laugh rather than the serious ones which bring the mood down.
- Go somewhere quiet and practice fake laughing. There is a branch of psychotherapy called laughter therapy which uses this technique. Strangely if you fake laugh loudly and for long enough you can actually make yourself laugh and still gain the benefits. I personally find the most exaggerated, fake, loud, ho-ho-ho laughter makes me laugh quickest. Experiment by yourself or even better with others to find the type of fake laughter that makes you laugh.
- Read some funny books or joke books for variety or even start learning to tell jokes to others.
- Set yourself homework to improve your positivity, optimism and gratefulness.

Chapter 12: Pineapple's - Bromelian

The other fantastic "apple" apart from the "golden apple" (tomato) already discussed is the pineapple (Ananus comosus). Fresh pineapple juice contains a range of fantastic nutrients such as manganese and vitamin C but of particular interest in the fight against cancer is the enzyme mixture, bromelain. Bromelain is a mixture of protein-digesting enzymes— cysteine proteinases which are often referred to as proteolytic enzymes or proteases. Bromelain is present in the flowering plant family called Bromeliaceae however the most well-known and farmed is the pineapple. Although present in the whole pineapple plant it found in higher concentrations in the stem. Pineapples have a long history of being used for medical purposes especially in South America and Germany and is still widely used as a meat tenderizer.

It is like a lot enzymes, a delicate protein that can be denatured or broken down by excessive heat or processing and so is probably best sourced for eating from fresh juice or fruit. Although clearly also like all proteins eaten it is likely to be substantially broken down during digestion by the body's own "digestive juices" (e.g. stomach acid and enzymes). It is thought by many if sufficient pineapple juice is consumed a small amount of bromelain will still be absorbed by the body. Bromelain is a proteolytic enzyme well known to the food industry because of its ability to break down proteins (especially fibrin and fibrinogen) and so hence its use as a meat tenderizer.

It had been shown that bromelain has an anti-inflammatory impact by physically removing cell surface molecules that are required for leucocytes to be activated and migrate. This anti-inflammatory impact of bromelain has been developed by researchers for the treatment of many immune-mediated diseases such as irritable bowel disease (IBD). There has been marked improvements in patients with severe colitis following ingestion of bromelain with decreased secretion of the pro-inflammatory substances known as cytokines and chemokines. Along with many other anti-inflammatory compounds, bromelain's anti-inflammatory properties seem to be equally wide reaching with benefits being noted in people with arthritis and osteoarthritis when it is used at the same time as trypsin and rutin.

An interesting research study on mice has shown that fresh pineapple juice has sufficient content of bromelain to have a therapeutic impact on their colitis, colitis-induced mortality and tumours present due to colitis. Bromelain has shown to have a beneficial impact on a wide range of cancers, but the research is still in its relatively early stages. However bromelain is an active enzyme and is like most proteins denatured by increased temperatures and so boiled pineapple juice as expected showed no therapeutic benefit. This would indicate that if consuming pineapple juice for this benefit that non-pasteurized fresh juice should be used. Although pill supplements are available it would seem to be less biologically active or absorbable so for longer term dietary supplementation the consumption of fresh unadulterated and unprocessed pineapple fruit would probably be more beneficial. Studies have shown previously frozen fresh pineapple juice still exerts an anti-inflammatory impact which not only can reduce colitis but also reduce the growth of inflammation-based new tumours in the colon. It is important to be aware that bromelain can increase heart rate and so if you suffer from heart disease additional care should be taken however I am unaware of reports of anyone dying as a result of drinking fresh pineapple in reasonable amounts for this reason!

Some of the most difficult cancerous tumours to beat are known as gliomas and are tumours of the nervous system. Primary brain tumours (gliomas) occur and generally stay in the central nervous system. They are often the most spread out throughout the tissue often making surgical removal and local radiotherapy poor methods of treatment due to the likely possibility of damaging surrounding healthy tissue. This damage to good brain or CNS tissue can obviously have serious impacts to long-term health and quality of life. Often these gliomas follow the feeding source (the blood vessels) like a line of willows follow the line of a river. This nature means that they can spread causing substantial damage throughout the brain as they grow.

Interestingly as a tumour grows, its cell surface receptors may also change with changes in its cell adhesion qualities this is to aid the growth of gliomas via a mixture of cell migration and invasion. It was this fact linked to the bromelain's impact on cell surface molecules and its other anti-inflammatory impacts which led to researchers investigating its impact on glioma cells and whether bromelain could stop or slow down the invasive capacity of the glioma cells. Although only cell based research (in vitro) and not in vivo their results proved that bromelain can reversibly inhibit glioma cell migration and invasion by its enzymic action. This in itself is a significant discovery but they also found bromelain also impacted on the cells signalling cascades which might help to reduce the replication process. This knowledge may help limit or stop malignant cells invading normal brain tissue and surgical removal less damaging. At the moment they are considering local infusion of bromelain (injecting the tumour) for speed and accuracy but there is no data to confirm or deny that bodily absorbed bromelain may not have a worthwhile impact on gliomas.

Bromelain has also been shown to have significant impacts on leukaemia and melanoma cells. One of its biggest impacts is its ability to inhibit phosphorylation and signalling in T cells. The inhibition of specific signalling pathways which are directly linked to cell's nucleus are likely to play an important part in reducing tumour cell growth and division. Of almost equal significance is bromelain's inhibition of cell adhesion which may also cause an inability of the cells to transmit signals normally thus leading to reduced protein synthesis within cells.

Jobs to do

1. Go to shop today and buy 5 cartons of fresh pineapple juice (unprocessed) and have at least a pint a day if not more to gain the full benefit. Like all increases in fruit juice gradually increase your body's tolerance to it, as a more sensitive stomach or bowel may react in the usual expressive ways!! Put it on your weekly shopping list so that it becomes part of your regular diet.

Chapter 13: Broccoli & Cruciferous Vegetables

It is widely known and accepted that high levels of vegetable intake are well connected to a lower risk of acquiring several types of cancers. Significant consumption of cruciferous vegetables in particular (e.g., broccoli, cabbage, cauliflower) are associated with a lower risk of cancers especially those of the colon, lung, prostate, cervix and breast.

Cruciferous vegetables are from the Cruciferae (aka Brassicaceae) family. They include many green leaf vegetables such as cress, kale and Brussel sprouts and are named in Latin after their cross-shaped four petal flowers. Cruciferous vegetables contain a variety of stimulating chemicals that appear to interact and reduce the carcinogenic process. One chemical of particular interest is indole-3-carbinol (I3C). Indole-3-carbinol, a common phytochemical in the human diet, is present in all members of the cruciferous vegetable family. I3C occurs naturally as a glucosinolate in cabbage, cauliflower, and broccoli. Over ten years ago I3C was found to inhibit tumour growth in animals given cancer inducing chemicals. Many more studies have shown the wide action of I3C's anticarcinogenic properties. Recently, it has become clear that I3C has the potential to prevent and even to treat a number of common cancers, especially those that are oestrogen related. It seems highly likely that the anticarcinogenesis of I3C is linked to the action of detoxification enzymes referred to as the cytochrome P-450 system.

Molecular studies suggest that variations in detoxification enzymes, particularly glutathione S-transferase may influence cancer risk in response to cruciferous vegetables. Indole-3-Carbinol is one of the most widely researched bioactive food components within cruciferous vegetables. This compound arises from indolyl–methyl glucosinolate when cruciferous vegetables are crushed or cooked. Eaten I3C can be converted into the bioactive chemical DIindolylMethane (DIM), within the gut. Since DIM accumulates in the cell nucleus, it seems possible that DIM is responsible for the cellular impacts that have been linked to I3C.

Several mechanisms may account for the anticancer properties of I3C/DIM including changes in cell cycle progression, apoptosis, and DNA repair. It remains unclear which chemical is the most responsible for the anticancer properties linked to cruciferous vegetables. There are many laboratory studies which provide evidence that I3C/ DIM can influence and possibly regulate to some degree both apoptosis and cell proliferation. Loss of cell cycle control is a well-recognized prevention to tumour development and proliferation. I3C has been shown to initiate interference with the cell cycle in tumours in human cancers. Tumour growth could also be reduced due to an increase in apoptosis.

NFkB as previously discussed is a transcription factor that has an important role in regulating the expression of genes involved with the apoptotic process. Recent research indicates that I3C modulates the apoptosis (programmed cell death) by inhibiting the activation of NFkB, which helps reduce significantly the activation of anti-apoptotic genes. Very small amounts of I3C can induce apoptosis in tumour cells within as little as 2 days with an increase reducing that time even further. It is still unclear if this interaction on NFkB production by I3C is a direct or indirect relationship but for it to affect such change so quickly in such small amounts would indicate that it is likely to be a signalling chemical or catalyst.

As previously discussed tumour growth is an unnatural rapid proliferation of cells, which requires large amounts of energy from the cell. This energy is obtained from the powerhouse of the cell its mitochondria. Increased energy production in the mitochondria can lead to an excess of potentially toxic oxidants due to oxidative stress. I3C might achieve its anti-cancer abilities due to its innate ability to interfere and stop the mitochondrial membrane potential, thus limiting cells mitochondrial-associated energy output.

I3C taken as a supplement (the equivalent of one third of a head of cabbage per day) reverses precancerous changes in women with up to stage III cervical dysplasia. A diet rich in cruciferous vegetables or I3C supplements causes regression of tumours, decreases their growth rates or re-occurrence in the majority of patients with recurrent laryngeal papillomatosis. Lab studies suggest that this phytochemical can act in several different ways to prevent cancer, as well as to selectively kill transformed cells.

I3C is rapidly converted in the stomach to a variety of other end products, but primarily DIindolylMethane (DIM). Interestingly plasma from humans and rats fed I3C contains no detectable I3C, but large amounts of DIM, as well as other metabolites. Thus DIM, rather than I3C, is probably the major compound initially available to cells after ingestion of I3C. I3C is also converted slowly to DIM at neutral pH, with the result that either compound is active in vitro. Lab results have shown that both I3C and DIM induce apoptosis in breast carcinoma cells.

There has been fairly extensive research using mice showing an impact on a range of tumours such as laryngeal, prostrate, breast and cervical cancers. Some researchers have shown I3C by mouth can in fact prevent the start of cervical cancer in those mice with human papillomavirus (HPV) oncogenes exposed to high levels of oestrogen. Normally these would go on to develop cervical cancer. It therefore seems reasonable to some degree to consider that one of the ways I3C works is by interfering with oestrogen metabolism by stimulating the cytochrome P450 system. Based on a range of studies it appears that this is not the only way that I3C impacts cancer cells.

Isothiocyanates have stimulated a lot of interest in research laboratories over the last thirty years because of their cancer fighting abilities in animals. A wide range of Isothiocyanates act in a chemo protective manner against different tumours caused by a range of chemical carcinogens. This quite strongly indicates that there is a consistent biological model relating to their impact. It is generally accepted that induction of cancer-protective Phase 2 enzymes (e.g. glutathione transferases, quinone reductase and glucuronosyltransferases) and/or inhibition of carcinogen-activating Phase 1 enzymes play a major role in this protection.

The Phase 2 enzymes are involved in oxidative stress management as discussed earlier. Nicotinamide Adenine Dinucleotide Phosphate, abbreviated $NADP^+$ is a coenzyme used in a wide range of key reactions including nucleic acid synthesis (a key component of a cell's DNA), which require NADPH as a reducing chemical. NADPH is the reduced form of $NADP^+$.

NADPH acts as a reducing agent for biosynthetic reactions and the redox reactions involved in protecting against the toxicity of oxidants or Reactive Oxygen Species (ROS). Although ROS have an important role in the human body to destroy pathogens via the very powerful oxidative burst process during inflammation they can also be highly toxic to the human body and carcinogenic if not managed by the body properly. The rise in the public's awareness of the importance of antioxidants generally is testament to the wide-ranging potential negative impacts of ROS

Isothiocyanates are present in edible plants, particularly in cruciferous vegetables (including woad famously used by tribes and clans from Great Britain for health, dying and possibly face paint). Isothiocyanates are widely consumed by humans in considerable quantities. It is increasingly clear that an increased vegetable-based diet intake is a key factor in cancer prevention and not just the reduction of red meats. When animal tissues are exposed to Isothiocyanates there is an induction of several Phase 2 enzymes such as glutathione transferases, quinone reductase and glucuronosyltransferases.

Isothiocyanates have been shown to block chemical carcinogenesis against a diverse group of carcinogens in many target tissues of several animal species in different ways. They also inhibit Phase 1 enzymes involved in carcinogen activation and induce Phase 2 enzymes that accelerate cellular disposal of activated carcinogens in a variety of cells and animal tissues.

The anticarcinogenic and the enzyme-regulating activities of Isothiocyanates have been shown to be concentration dependent but that the most desirable level for action has yet to be fully determined due to the high number of other variables.

More research as always is indicated but in particular the accumulation of Isothiocyanates within cells and Isothiocyanates complex relationship with phase 2 detoxification enzymes, especially glutathione transferases and NADPH, needs significant understanding. These phase 2 detoxification enzymes are an essential component of the body's regulation of toxic and carcinogenic chemicals.

In conclusion, I3C and DIM from the natural foods of the family Cruciferae exert significant anticancer effects mediated through the regulation of the cell cycle, cell proliferation, apoptosis, oncogenesis, transcription, and cell-signal transduction (e.g. NFkB & MAPK.)

Jobs to do

1. Go to a shop today and regularly to buy enough cruciferous vegetables especially broccoli to have significant amounts twice a day (lunch and dinner). Ideally you should eat at least half a large broccoli head every day. Remember if you have a delicate stomach which isn't used to too receiving high levels of vegetable matter you should build up to this slowly or you may have an "explosion" (both air and liquid) to deal with in the bowel department!

2. Stop buying so much meat especially red meats from now on you should have a very low intake of meat and replace it with other sources of proteins such as beans, nuts and lentils.

3. Buy indole-3-carbinol supplements and take as directed

Remember all advice is given assuming that you have consulted and sought agreement with your doctor and that you and you alone are responsible for anything which you willingly put in your body!

Chapter 14: Homeopathic Condurango, Arsenicum Album & Ruta Graveolens

There has been renewed significant interest in investigating different plants and compounds used by homeopathic doctors for centuries and others to identify effective ingredients using modern chemical and molecular methods. For example, many antitumor drugs in current clinical use, such as podophyllotoxins, diosmetins, and taxanes are taken from plants.

However this chapter will focus on three heavily researched ones, in particular those that have been used in cases of cancer in homeopathic dilutions.

With the significant side-effects of some traditional medicines, people are looking towards alternative medicines with fewer and less toxic side-effects to complement their treatment plans. Homeopathy has become a major complementary and alternative medicine in many countries today. In homeopathy, micro doses of very high dilutions (potentized) of natural substances are generally preferred over tinctures (crude extracts). The initial drug substance is generally dissolved in an aqueous solution of alcohol (often 70%) and is potentized in gradual steps of dilution with agitation known as sucussion. On a centesimal scale, when 1 mL of tincture is diluted with 99 mL of an aqueous solution of ethanol and given 10 sucussions (mechanical shakes) a potency 1C is produced. When 1 mL of 1C is again diluted with 99 mL of an aqueous solution of alcohol and given 10 sucussions, the potency 2C is produced, and so on. This potentizing and diluting process means when the drug has attained potency 12C, it has been diluted to 10^{-24} (beyond Avogadro's limit), and thus the existence of a single molecule of the original drug substance becomes highly improbable. Although some researchers have demonstrated the existence of nanoparticles of the original drug in such ultra-highly diluted homeopathic drugs, the efficacy is often questioned by researchers as to the precise mechanism of drug action which has still not been firmly established. This has not stopped some researchers review, revisiting and testing homeopathic drugs especially in countries where homeopathy is a key part of the healthcare system such as India or Germany for example. Condurango (*Marsdenia condurango*) is a key homeopathic remedy which has been used for centuries by homeopaths in the treatment of cancer with some homeopaths claiming great success in many cases.

Homeopathy is not so widely used in China but they have used herbal medicine in similar ways as part of Traditional Chinese Medicine (TCM) in the battle against cancer. *Marsdenia tenacissima* is a biological relative in the same family as Condurango and is also a perennial climber that is native in the highlands of Nepal, Yunnan and Guizhou Provinces of China.

The dried stems of *Marsdenia tenacissima* are also known as "Tong-guang-teng". The plant is present in the pharmacopeia of the People's Republic of China and has been used in TCM for thousands of years for a range of ailments including tumours. This ancient plant and its medicinal effect are noted as far back as the Ming Dynasty. Modern lab studies have shown that it has not only anti-tumour effects but also protects the liver and induces immunomodulatory effects. Many steroidal glycosides have been identified from it including tenacissoside, marsdenoside and tenacigenoside. A medical treatment regime containing it as the active ingredient has been available and regulated in the Chinese healthcare system for many years to be used alone or combined with radiotherapy or chemotherapy for cancer treatment.

Interestingly for our British readers it is a mark of the interconnectedness of life or just strange coincidence, that a genus of plants with anti-tumour properties is named after a famous Marsden in London from the 1800s. It was named after William Marsden, the avid plant collector, pioneer in the scientific study of Indonesia and the first secretary of the Admiralty during the successful Battle of Trafalgar and not the other famous unrelated Marsden from the 1800s, William Marsden, surgeon, whose wife died of cancer, leading to him being inspired to focus on new treatments and "battle" cancer and so form the world famous anti-cancer hospital the Royal Marsden Hospital.

The dried bark of Condurango (*Marsdenia condurango*), belonging to Asclepiadaceae family. It is also known as the Condor plant as it is native to Peru and the Andes and inhabits the highlands and is synonymous with the ancient power associated with the bird. Although it has been used for a wide range of cancers Condurango has often be used against a variety of breast, digestive problems and oesophageal cancer.

Condurango is known to contain conduritol and other unique glycosides. It is believed, that the biologically active component of Condurango, conduritol, is a potent anti-tumour agent. Unfortunately the molecular mechanism of its specific anti-tumour activity is still unclear. In lab and animal studies the ability of the alcoholic extract of Condurango is proved to induce cytotoxicity and apoptosis in several non-small-cell lung cancer cell lines and in lung cancer of rats. There have been no randomized controlled trials of homeopathic Condurango on humans but many homeopathic individual case reviews.

Arsenic Trioxide is a highly powerful and toxic substance which has been used by poisoners throughout history due to its deathly toxicity and limited taste. However it has also been used in highly diluted form by ancient Chinese medicine and western homeopaths down the centuries to stimulate healing and in its medicinal form is called Arsenicum Album. Although homeopathy is not widely supported by traditional medicine as clinically beneficial in the UK, it is better supported by many European and global countries such as Germany, France, Iran, India & Brazil. It was and is often used in severe ill health cases where there are symptoms of diarrhoea, vomiting, stomach cramps and nervousness. These symptoms often appear in the later stages of many cancers and when they are present it is believed that the homeopathic remedy will be most beneficial. However many homeopaths also recommend it before these symptoms present as part of a prophylactic approach. Most will recommend a low potency (e.g. 12C) so as to stimulate the body to self-heal in a gradual fashion. It is generally advisable to take homeopathic remedies under the guidance of a trained homeopath rather than "self-treat", although many people do "treat" themselves.

Renewed scientific interest in this chemical has taken place in the field of cancer care on discovery of its ability to cause apoptosis (programmed cell death) and cell growth inhibition. Arsenic Trioxide is an ancient drug that has been recognized to act directly on cancer cell mitochondria. Dysfunction of apoptosis has been linked with many serious diseases including cancer. A good example of this dysfunction of apoptosis being a significant factor is its involvement in the start of chronic lymphocytic leukaemia and some lymphomas, some multiple myeloma cells, and some solid tumour cells including oesophageal cancer and neuroblastoma cells.

One recent scientific study in China showed that Arsenic Trioxide in low doses actually exerted substantial growth inhibition in all malignant lymphocytic cells examined. There were also significant examples of decreased cell viability leading to apoptosis. In short it was found extremely low concentrations or high dilutions of Arsenic trioxide are levels which are tolerated by patients can inhibit growth, proliferation and often can induce apoptosis in cancerous cells especially lymphocytes and those of lymphomas.

Clearly for reasons of its toxicity Arsenic Trioxide is not freely available but homeopathic dilutions/potencies of Arsenicum Album are available which may exert similar influence on cancerous cells. It is widely accepted that homeopathic dilutions of 12C & above are unlikely to contain an actual molecule of Arsenic Trioxide and so the mechanism of homeopathy's action is still far from understood or accepted but it may be considered as part of your complementary approach.

Ruta Graveolens is commonly known as Rue or Herb of Grace and is an herbaceous perennial originally from the Mediterranean. It has spread its natural habitat throughout Europe and the world most likely due to man's historical use of this plant. It is now so common that many countries consider it a weed although other countries actively grow it. Rue has been among the key plants of the European medical pharmacy since ancient times. Its curative action has been recorded by medical leaders such as Hippocrates, Dioscorides and Pliny. It is part of the Rutaceae and has many active components including rutin. Its medicinal value was considered so great that rue was taken and introduced to North, Central and South America, China, India, Middle East and South Africa.

Ruta Graveolens extract has been used in the past to aid healing and treatment for a wide variety of illnesses and diseases such as eye problems, rheumatism, dermatitis, pain and many inflammatory diseases. Its anti-inflammatory, anti-diabetic, antibacterial, antifungal, insecticide and antihistamine properties are most likely its key benefits in the fight against cancer. The pure extract is very powerful and has a significant impact on the central nervous system. It acts as a poison in large doses causing excessive irritation of the gut and tongue with vertigo, reduced mental ability, tremors, liver and kidney damage and even death. The extract has many different alkaloids, coumarins, terpenoids, flavonoids and furoquinolines. The extract contains a very wide number of other chemicals, including saponin, tannins, glycosides, and the key active flavonoids, rutin and quercetin.

The extract when applied topically has helped with a wide range of inflammatory and oxidative stress problems such as oedema and arthritis. Clearly its extract in its pure form should never be taken by mouth, but at homeopathic dilutions and potencies above 12C it has been used safely. Some patients with gliomas have had better results when using Ruta in homeopathic dilutions in a complementary manner than those who have not. Ruta in homeopathic dilutions appears to have a negative impact on cancer cells by preventing further carcinogenesis and by protecting normal B-lymphoid cells against hydrogen peroxide-induced chromosomal damage. Ruta has been found to have anti-tumour activity in the lab using mammals. Research using human breast cancer cells has also shown that Ruta extract has the power to reduce cell growth and stimulate cell death. It has been found that at homeopathic dilutions or low concentrations that Ruta extract activates the inhibition of lipid peroxidation, activates the p53 or tumour suppressor gene pathway and also activates the caspase pathway. All of these activations have a direct or indirect impact on apoptosis or programmed cell death of cancer cells. Many of these pathways are sulphur and cysteine dependent so a diet which contains a healthy level of these may also be beneficial in combination.

These two remedies have had some scientific study by non-homeopaths but there are a wide range of homeopathic remedies that have been linked by homeopaths to help holistically in the fight against cancer but very few significant randomised or controlled scientific trials to help give the scientific rigour desired by traditional medicine. It is considered by most homeopaths for homeopathy to be most effective that it is individualised and therefore a consultation with a trained homeopath is what they recommend. It is now possible to do telephone of video-call homeopathic consultations using WhatsApp or FaceTime etc. Non-homeopaths and most reputable homeopaths would recommend that no traditional treatment is stopped unless agreed by your oncologist.

Jobs to do

- Consider getting Condurango, Arsenicum Album & Ruta Graveolens homeopathic remedies (potency 12C or 30C) from your traditional pharmacist if available or homeopathic pharmacy or apothecary (www.homeopathic-apothecary.com) and discussing their use with your oncologist etc. Be aware that many homeopaths would not recommend this combination and non-individualised approach.

- Consider consulting a registered homeopath in a holistic integrated manner with your oncologist. (http://www.homeopathyservices.co.uk) or (https://facultyofhomeopathy.org/find-a-homeopath)

Chapter 15: Turmeric, Black Pepper & Red Chilli Peppers

Turmeric is commonly used as a spice and contains many important chemicals. A key one is curcumin. The most important chemical components of turmeric are a group of compounds called curcuminoids, which include curcumin, demethoxycurcumin, and bisdemethoxycurcumin. The most-studied compound is curcumin, which constitutes approximately 3% of powdered turmeric. In addition, other important components include turmerone, atlantone, and zingiberene.

Turmeric comes from drying and grinding the roots of *Curcuma longa*. The lipid-soluble yellow chemical which comes from the curcuma plants is used for cooking, cosmetics, and textile dying. In the 1400s, turmeric was available in European markets provided by Middle Eastern traders. Turmeric and the isolated curcumin are used now mainly as colorants in many food products. Turmeric is a key ingredient of curry powder.

Turmeric shows many health benefits by acting in an anti-inflammatory, antioxidant, antiviral, and anti-infectious manner. These and other properties help it to enhance the healing of wounds and ulcers. In recent years there has been increased scientific interest in curcumin for treatment or prevention of cancer with a significant increase in research papers.

It has been shown that curcumin by itself or in combination with other drugs increases cell death in a wide range of cancer tumour cells, including brain tumours, sarcoma, breast cancer, ovarian cancer, testicular cancer, prostate cancer, pancreatic cancer, liver cancer, biliary cancer, gastric cancer, colorectal cancer, lung cancer, mesothelioma, renal cancer, bladder cancer, head and neck cancer, and lymphomas. Many lab and *in vivo* studies with turmeric show consistent impacts including suppression and reversal of cancers.

Some studies tend to indicate that curcumin's anticarcinogenic action occurs due to its negative impact on arachidonic acid metabolism. The cyclo-oxygenase (COX) enzyme speeds up the production of prostaglandins (PGs) from arachidonic acid. There are at least two types of this enzyme known as COX-1 & COX-2. They initially at first glance appeared to have antagonist impacts. COX-1 being involved in normal physiologic function and its associated PGs playing a protective role, whilst the other, COX-2, being stimulated often by carcinogenic promotors such as toxins and oncogenes. COX-2 was and is in fact found present in many different tumours and is connected with carcinogenesis and angiogenesis. Although this knowledge has stimulated much research and interest in COX-2 along the lines of believing its relationship to be straightforward and a direct cause of cancer, there has been little benefit with anti-COX-2 drug therapy. One study of a so-called COX-2-selective inhibitor drug was indeed stopped due to its serious side-effects.

Studies of COX-1 have noted its involvement in angiogenesis (development of a blood supply which many quickly growing cancers needs) and so a similar approach this time for COX-1 inhibitors is being examined. Curcumin and chemical equivalents are showing significant inhibitory effects on COX-1 activity.

Curcumin seems to induce death of cancer cells by activation of apoptosis pathways. This activation of apoptosis by curcumin occurs with modulation of multiple signalling pathways. It appears curcumin acts differently depending on the cancer type with activation and or inhibition of certain signalling pathways resulting in cell death via different routes. This is quite unusual for a single substance and so has stimulated a lot of research across cancer types. Curcumin has also been shown to modulate telomerase which enables cancer cells to die. It seems that curcumin can impact cancer cells whilst have limited or no toxic effects on healthy cells. It is not just researchers that are aware of the benefits of curcumin but also clinicians and patients are using it more widely as it appears to also enhance standard chemotherapy treatments. However care should be taken as curcumin interacts with a wide range of drugs in different ways.

Of even more interest is that curcumin has been seen to stop or interfere with cancer cell movement via its invasion or metastasis process. A key step in tumour metastasis is the process of epithelial cell change usually accompanied by a reduction in an epithelial gene being expressed (cadherin - CDH1). These CDH1 genes require Calcium ions to function but also can be stimulated by curcumin which has been noted by researchers to arrest this epithelial change process. Another stimulus which seems to increase the cell motility in cancer cells is lysophosphatidic acid (LPA). It has also been noted that curcumin can also reduce this LPA stimulus and thus reduce cancer cell motility. These two effects alone help to show that curcumin does not only reduce tumour growth but also metastasis formation in many types of cancer.

It has also been seen using cell and animal studies that curcumin and its derivatives can also reduce or slow tumour formation in many different tumours. Curcumin significantly inhibited the formation of cancer tumours or pre-cancerous lesions in animal models for breast, liver, gastric and colon cancers when the controls with no curcumin treatment evolved significant cancers. The regulatory activity of curcumin seems to be responsible at least to some degree for such cancer prevention and also appear to control some bacterial growth such as *Helicobacter pylori*.

The anti-cancer impacts of vitamin D have been noted by many researchers, but data also suggests that for some cancer types, sunlight can reduce cancer risk independent from vitamin D. Importantly curcumin increases cancer cell death and differentiation of vitamin D-treated tumour cells. The interaction and direct attaching of curcumin to vitamin D receptors has been seen.

Curcumin can lower the number of myeloid-derived suppressor cells, which are have an important role in immuno-suppression of cancer cells. People with cancer often have a dysfunction of the immune system caused or directly related to the tumour cells. Research indicates that curcumin is able to improve the immune function in animals with cancer. Curcumin as an anti-inflammatory chemical can suppress T cells. The balance between immune-stimulation and immuno-suppression might be related to the concentration of curcumin. This is of interest because in some cancers the relationship with the immune system can be very complicated. This is because not only do cytotoxic T cells kill cancer cells, but the T cells can also provide survival support for cancer cells.

There are a number of other impacts that curcumin has on cells which have been explored that may have important effects on cancers and their progression. These include that curcumin can suppress certain enzymes (histone deacetylases) and can slow or stop DNA methylation. For some cancer cells both these activities (DNA methylation or histone deacetylation) are very important in gene expression and cancer cells susceptibility to cytotoxic drugs. Another reason for taking seriously the power of curcumin is that it has been shown to interfere with the transcription/duplication process by the Human Immunodeficiency Virus (HIV- type 1). It is being further investigated if curcumin can modulate the activity of endogenous retroviruses (ERV) in certain cancer cells. It has been found in some tumours that there are a high number of viruses such as Epstein Barr Virus (EBV).

Curcumin can slow or stop B cell immortalization caused by EBV and in fact significant cancer cell death appears to occur in the presence of curcumin. It also seems apparent that also general oxidative stress promotes B cell immortalization by EBV. It is therefore a possibility that the anti-oxidant activity of curcumin might inhibit this, just like it has been seen with vitamin E.

The standard pharmaceutical approach to try to find the active component and then mass produce on an industrial scale can often miss subtle interaction between components and this might be the case with curcumin and turmeric. Another interesting question that remains to be addressed is whether the effects of turmeric are only mediated by curcumin or whether additional turmeric ingredients are involved. Some recent research helps to confirm this hypothesis by suggesting that curcumin-free turmeric extracts also have cancer preventing activities with noticeable differences between turmeric's and curcumin's action on pro-inflammatory genes.

The human body's ability to digest and then absorb curcumin is not as effective as is desirable due to rapid metabolism and excretion. Curcumin is rapidly processed by the intestines and liver and thus limiting the curcumin available for the body to use. Studies have shown that when curcumin is taken in conjunction with piperine (the active ingredient in black pepper) that the body is able to absorb more curcumin. Not only does piperine have this effect but these polyphenols, curcumin and piperine have been seen to be able to limit the growth of malignant breast cells.

Pepper & The Immune System

This often overlooked condiment is in fact probably one of the original superfoods which has helped people over the centuries. A review of its long history of use shows it widely respected and valued so that it was once even referred to as "Black gold". **The polyphenol piperine is isolated from black and long peppers. Piperine has been reported to reduce lung cancer incidence.** The alcoholic extract of the fruits of the pepper plant (*Piper longum*) and its main active component called piperine have been researched with regards to their immunomodulatory and anti-tumour activity. Piperine is also present in black pepper. The Alcoholic extract of the fruits is most significant because even with very low levels it effectively killed lymphoma cells and Ehrlich carcinoma cells. Piperine is also noted to be cytotoxic towards these cells. Research on mice has proved remarkable with the *Piper longum* extract and piperine increasing total White Blood Cells count to 142.8% and 138.9% respectively. This is a very significant increase and highly useful in the fight against cancer.

Capsaicin is a key active ingredient present in hot green and red chilli peppers of the Capsicum family and is a widely used ingredient for cooking. Its analgesic and anti-inflammatory properties have also meant that it is widely used topically as well as in clinical practice for the treatment of a variety of pain conditions. However although used medically for centuries for general complaints more recently capsaicin is also recognized for its pharmacological and toxicological properties in the treatment of cancer.

Large research studies have shown that capsaicin can promote or prevent carcinogenic activities both in the test-tube and humans. Large scale epidemiological studies indicate that capsaicin consumption may reduce the risk of colon cancer but excessive consumption appears to irritate the stomach lining significantly and cause cancer. Even though there has been decades of cancer-related research, the exact nature of how capsaicin works is not fully understood. Many researchers believe that its anti-cancer action is not related to its analgesic action in sensory neurons but more likely that it limits Vascular Endothelial Growth Factor (VEGF)-induced angiogenesis or in other words it limits the growth of new blood vessels to "feed" the growing tumour. Capsaicin also appears to impede cell division through the regulation of cyclin. It is interesting to note that other anti-angiogenic chemicals such as such as endostatin and curcumin also suppress Retinoblastoma protein phosphorylation and DNA synthesis of endothelial cells through down-regulation of cyclin.

Animal research has shown that capsaicin significantly limits tumour growth. This has included directly injecting capsaicin into skin tumours as well as including in the diets of rodents with cancers. It has been noticed that it has its anti-angiogenesis effect without affecting healthy blood vessels already present.

In general how bio-available capsaicin is after eating red chilli pepper or how bio-available piperine and pepper extract is following normal intake is not fully understood. It is understood though that piperine does reduce the human liver enzyme CYP3A4 and P-glycoprotein along with other enzymes important in cell detoxification. These include the CYP450 enzymes which have multiple key functions. This is important because just as grapefruit can interfere with the effectiveness of certain drugs by interfering with CYP450 enzymes, so can piperine and thus pepper extract, therefore as with everything noted in this book all things should be discussed with you doctor before considering in a complementary manner. **This being understood, piperine can improve the absorption of curcumin by up to 2000% in humans most probably by its interaction with liver enzymes.** The combined power of turmeric and pepper extract has been shown to be highly significant in cancer growth prevention in animals. Of benefit in the fight against cancer piperine, has also shown intriguing impacts on cognitive function and having an almost anti-depressant quality.

Jobs to do

- Create your own alcoholic extract for turmeric and black pepper using vodka and take a small shot daily following consultation with your doctor.

- Be careful with red chilli peppers as some people can have a powerful reaction to them, but try to slowly increase in your diet if you do not already.

- If not make your own favourite curry with ample helpings of turmeric, chilli and black pepper and have a curry a day once your digestive system can handle this regularly otherwise you may suffer the unpleasant and potentially debilitating consequences of too much curry! This is far from ideal if trying to maintain your weight.

I hope you find the information outlined useful as well as interesting. Hopefully it will stimulate wider debate about cancer and its treatment. Often complementary care or treatment is considered of minimal benefit and not scientific in its basis. I hope that by reviewing the scientific references detailed in the next few pages for you that your discussions with your doctor help to re-balance this. The scientific papers reviewed are from highly respected and esteemed, peer-reviewed journals which both you and your doctor can access for more detail if required.

Finally all that remains is for me to wish you good luck in your fight against cancer.

Chapter 1: References

Ahmed H U (2009). The index lesion and the origin of prostate cancer. N Engl J Med. 2009;361:1704-1706.

Brenner DJ, Curtis RE, Hall EJ, Ron E. (2000). Second malignancies in prostate carcinoma patients after radiotherapy compared with surgery. Cancer. Jan 15;88(2):398-406.

Hall EJ, Wuu CS. (2003) Radiation-induced second cancers: the impact of 3D-CRT and IMRT. *Int J Radiat Oncol Biol Phys.*;56:83-88.

Lomax AJ, Boehringer T, Coray A, et al. (2001). Intensity modulated proton therapy: a clinical example. *Med Phys.*;28:317-324.

Lomax AJ, Pedroni E, Rutz H, Goitein G. (2004). The clinical potential of intensity modulated proton therapy. *Z Med Phys.*;14:147-152

Mock U, Georg D, Bogner J, Auberger T, Pötter R (2004). Treatment planning comparison of conventional, 3D conformal, and intensity-modulated photon (IMRT) and proton therapy for paranasal sinus carcinoma. Int J Radiat Oncol Biol Phys. Jan 1;58(1):147-54.

Ramaekers BL, Pijls-Johannesma M, Joore MA, van den Ende P, Langendijk JA, Lambin P, Kessels AG, Grutters JP. (2011). Systematic review and meta-analysis of radiotherapy in various head and neck cancers: Comparing photons, carbon-ions and protons. Cancer Treat Rev. May;37(3):185-201.

Trofimov A, Bortfeld T. (2003). Optimization of beam parameters and treatment planning for intensity modulated proton therapy. *Technol Cancer Res Treat.*;2:437-444.

Trofimov A, Paul L. Nguyen P L, M.D., Coen J J, Doppke K , Schneider R, Adams J, Bortfeld T, Zietman T, DeLaney T, Shipley W. (2007). Radiotherapy treatment of early stage prostate cancer with IMRT and protons: a treatment planning comparison. *Int. J. Radiat. Oncol. Biol. Phys.*;69(2):444.

Vargas C, Fryer A, Mahajan C, Indelicato D, Horne D, Chellini A, McKenzie C, Lawlor P, Henderson R, Li Z, Lin L, Olivier K, Keole S. (2008). Dose-volume comparison of proton therapy and intensity-modulated radiotherapy for prostate cancer. Int J Radiat Oncol Biol Phys. Mar 1;70(3):744-51.

Weber DC, Lomax AJ, Rutz HP, et al. (2004). Spot-scanning proton radiation therapy for recurrent, residual or untreated intracranial meningiomas. *Radiother Oncol.*. 71:251-258.

Weber DC, Trofimov AV, Delaney TF, Bortfeld T. (2004). A treatment planning comparison of intensity modulated photon and proton therapy for paraspinal sarcomas. *Int J Radiat Oncol Biol Phys.*;58:1596-1606.

Weber DC, Rutz HP, Pedroni ES, et al. (2005). Results of spot-scanning proton radiation therapy for chordoma and chondrosarcoma of the skull base: the Paul Scherrer Institut experience. *Int J Radiat Oncol Biol Phys.*;63:401-409.

Chapter 2: References

Peeters PH, Keinan-Boker L, van der Schouw YT, Grobbee DE. Phytoestrogens and breast cancer risk. Review of the epidemiological evidence. Breast Cancer Res Treat 2003; 77:171–183.

Petrakis NL, Barnes S, King EB, et al. Stimulatory influence of soy protein isolate on breast secretion in pre- and postmenopausal women. Cancer Epidemiol Biomarkers Prev 1996; 5:785–794.

Wojtaszek CA, Kochis LM, Cunningham RS. Nutrition impact symptoms in the oncology patient. Oncology Issues 2002; 17:15–17.

Deitel M, To TB. Major intestinal complications of radiotherapy. Management and nutrition. Arch Surg 1987; 122:1421–1424.

Ravasco P, Monteiro-Grillo I, Vidal PM, Camilo ME. Dietary counseling improves patient outcomes: a prospective, randomized, controlled trial in colorectal cancer patients undergoing radiotherapy. J Clin Oncol 2005; 23:1431–1438.

Rock CL. Dietary counseling is beneficial for the patient with cancer. J Clin Oncol 2005; 23:1348–1349.

Tohill BC, Seymour J, Serdula M, et al. What epidemiologic studies tell us about the relationship between fruit and vegetable consumption and body weight. Nutr Rev 2004; 62:365–374.

Slavin J. Why whole grains are protective: biological mechanisms. Proc Nutr Soc 2003; 62:129–134.

Rock CL, Flatt SW, Natarajan L, et al. Plasma carotenoids and recurrence-free survival in women with a history of breast cancer. J Clin Oncol 2005; 23:6631–6638.

Smith-Warner SA, Spiegelman D, Yaun SS, et al. Alcohol and breast cancer in women: a pooled analysis of cohort studies. JAMA 1998; 279:535–540.

Prasad KN, Kumar A, Kochupillai V, Cole WC. High doses of multiple antioxidant vitamins: essential ingredients in improving the efficacy of standard cancer therapy. J Am Coll Nutr 1999; 18:13–25.

Smith MR. Diagnosis and management of treatment-related osteoporosis in men with prostate carcinoma. Cancer 2003; 97(Suppl):789–795

Schmitz KH, Holtzman J, Courneya KS, et al. Controlled physical activity trials in cancer survivors: a systematic review and meta-analysis. Cancer Epidemiol Biomarkers Prev 2005; 14:1588–1595.

Knols R, Aaronson NK, Uebelhart D, et al. Physical exercise in cancer patients during and after medical treatment: a systematic review of randomized and controlled clinical trials. J Clin Oncol 2005; 23:3830–3842.

Jones LW, Eves ND, Courneya KS, et al. Effects of exercise training on antitumor efficacy of doxorubicin in MDA-MB-231 breast cancer xenografts. Clin Cancer Res 2005; 11:6695–6698.

Meyerhardt JA, Giovannucci EL, Holmes MD, et al. Physical activity and survival after colorectal cancer diagnosis. J Clin Oncol 2006; 24:3527–3534.

Ottery FD. Definition of standardized nutritional assessment and interventional pathways in oncology. Nutrition 1996; 12(Suppl):S15–S19.

Von Roenn JH. Pharmacologic interventions for cancer-related weight loss. Oncology Issues 2002; 17:18–21.

Kolonel LN. Fat, meat, and prostate cancer. Epidemiol Rev 2001; 23:72–81.

Sandhu MS, White IR, McPherson K. Systematic review of the prospective cohort studies on meat consumption and colorectal cancer risk: a meta-analytical approach. Cancer Epidemiol Biomarkers Prev 2001; 10:439–446.

World Cancer Research Fund/American Institute for Cancer Research. Food, nutrition, and the prevention of cancer: a global perspective. Washington, DC: American Institute for Cancer Research; 1997.

Joint WHO/FAO Expert Consultation on Diet, Nutrition and the Prevention of Chronic Diseases. Diet, Nutrition and the Prevention of Chronic Diseases: Report of a Joint WHO/FAO Expert Consultation. Geneva, Switzerland: World Health Organization; 2003.

Gogos CA, Ginopoulos P, Salsa B, et al. Dietary omega-3 polyunsaturated fatty acids plus vitamin E restore immunodeficiency and prolong survival for severely ill patients with generalized malignancy: a randomized control trial. Cancer 1998; 82:395–402.

Hardman WE. (n-3) fatty acids and cancer therapy. J Nutr 2004; 134(Suppl):3427S–3430S.

Monsen ER. Dietary reference intakes for the antioxidant nutrients: vitamin C, vitamin E, selenium, and carotenoids. J Am Diet Assoc 2000; 100:637–640.

Institute of Medicine, Food and Nutrition Board. Dietary Reference Intakes for Vitamin C, Vitamin E, Selenium, and Carotenoids. Washington, DC: National Academy Press; 2000.

Institute of Medicine, Food and Nutrition Board. Dietary Reference Intakes for Calcium, Phosphorus, Magnesium, Vitamin D, and Fluoride. Washington, DC: National Academy Press; 1997.

Institute of Medicine, Food and Nutrition Board. Dietary Reference Intakes for Thiamin, Riboflavin, Niacin, Vitamin B6, Folate, Vitamin B12, Panothenic Acid, Biotin, and Choline. Washington, DC: National Academy Press; 1998.

Labriola D, Livingston R. Possible interactions between dietary antioxidants and chemotherapy. Oncology (Williston Park) 1999; 13:1003–1008; discussion 1008, 1011–1012.

Lamson DW, Brignall MS. Antioxidants in cancer therapy; their actions and interactions with oncologic therapies. Altern Med Rev 1999; 4:304–329.

Chapter 3: References

Milner JA. Garlic: Its anticarcinogenic and antitumorigenic properties. Nutrition Reviews1996; 54:S82–S86.

Ross SA, Finley JW, Milner JA. Allyl sulfur compounds from garlic modulate aberrant crypt formation. Journal of Nutrition 2006; 136(3 Suppl):852S–854S.

Amagase H, Petesch BL, Matsuura H, Kasuga S, Itakura Y. Intake of garlic and its bioactive components. Journal of Nutrition 2001; 131(3s):955S–962S.

Fleischauer AT, Arab L. Garlic and cancer: A critical review of the epidemiologic literature. Journal of Nutrition 2001; 131(3s):1032S–1040S.

Gonzalez CA, Pera G, Agudo A, et al. Fruit and vegetable intake and the risk of stomach and oesophagus adenocarcinoma in the European Prospective Investigation into Cancer and Nutrition (EPIC-EURGAST). International Journal of Cancer 2006; 118(10): 2559–2566.

Steinmetz KA, Kushi LH, Bostick RM, Folsom AR, Potter JD. Vegetables, fruit, and colon cancer in the Iowa Women's Health Study. American Journal of Epidemiology 1994; 139(1):1–15.

Gao CM, Takezaki T, Ding JH, Li MS, Tajima K. Protective effect of allium vegetables against both esophageal and stomach cancer: A simultaneous case-referent study of a high-epidemic area in Jiangsu Province, China. Japanese Journal of Cancer Research1999; 90(6):614–621.

Setiawan VW, Yu GP, Lu QY, et al. Allium vegetables and stomach cancer risk in China.Asian Pacific Journal of Cancer Prevention 2005; 6(3):387–395.

Chan JM, Wang F, Holly EA. Vegetable and fruit intake and pancreatic cancer in a population-based case-control study in the San Francisco bay area. Cancer Epidemiology Biomarkers & Prevention 2005; 14(9):2093–2097.

Challier B, Perarnau JM, Viel JF. Garlic, onion and cereal fibre as protective factors for breast cancer: A French case-control study. European Journal of Epidemiology 1998; 14(8):737–747.

Li H, Li HQ, Wang Y, et al. An intervention study to prevent gastric cancer by micro-selenium and large dose of allitridum. Chinese Medical Journal (English) 2004; 117(8):1155–1160.

Tanaka S, Haruma K, Kunihiro M, et al. Effects of aged garlic extract (AGE) on colorectal adenomas: A double-blinded study. Hiroshima Journal of Medical Sciences 2004; 53(3–4):39–45.

Tilli CM, Stavast-Kooy AJ, Vuerstaek JD, et al. The garlic-derived organosulfur component ajoene decreases basal cell carcinoma tumor size by inducing apoptosis. Archives of Dermatological Research 2003; 295(3):117–123.

Ruddock PS, Liao M, Foster BC, et al. Garlic natural health products exhibit variable constituent levels and antimicrobial activity against Neisseria gonorrhoeae, Staphylococcus aureus and Enterococcus faecalis. Phytotherapy Research 2005; 19(4):327–334.

L'vova GN, Zasukhina GD. Modification of repair DNA synthesis in mutagen-treated human fibroblasts during adaptive response and the antimutagenic effect of garlic extract. Genetika 2002; 38(3):306–309.

Visioli F, Galli C, Plasmati E, Hernandez A, Colombo C, Sala A. Olive phenol hydroxytyrosol prevents passive smoking-induced oxidative stress. Circulation. 2000; 102: 2169–2171.

Cecil R. Pace-Asciak, Olga Rounova, Susan E. Hahn[b], Eleftherios P. Diamandis and David M. Goldberg (1996). Wines and grape juices as modulators of platelet aggregation in healthy human subjects. Clinica Chimica Acta Volume 246, Issues 1-2, Pages 163-182.

Coccia A, Mosca L, Puca R, Mangino G, Rossi A, Lendaro E. (2016). Extra-virgin olive oil phenols block cell cycle progression and modulate chemotherapeutic toxicity in bladder cancer cells. Oncol Rep. Oct 5. 10.3892/.2016.5150.

Wallerath T, Deckert G, Ternes T, Anderson H, Li H, Witte K, Forstermann U. Resveratrol, a polyphenolic phytoalexin present in red wine, enhances expression and activity of endothelial nitric oxide synthase. Circulation. 2002; 106: 1652–1658.

Kris-Etherton P, Eckel RH, Howard BV, St Jeor S, Bazzarre TL. Lyon Diet Heart Study: Benefits of a Mediterranean-Style, National Cholesterol Education Program/American Heart Association Step I Dietary Pattern on Cardiovascular Disease. Ciculation. 2001; 103: 1823–1825.

Visioli F, Bellomo G, Galli C. Free radical-scavenging properties of olive oil polyphenols. Biochem Biophys Res Commun. 1998; 247: 60–64.

Miller NJ, Rice-Evans CA. Antioxidant activity of resveratrol in red wine. Clin Chem. 1995; 41: 1789–1794.

Bertelli A, Bertelli AA, Gozzini A, Giovannini L. Plasma and tissue resveratrol concentrations and pharmacological activity. Drugs Exp Clin Res. 1998; 24: 133–138.

Visioli F, Galli C, Plasmati E, Hernandez A, Colombo C, Sala A. Olive phenol hydroxytyrosol prevents passive smoking-induced oxidative stress. Circulation. 2000; 102: 2169–2171.

Frankel E, Waterhouse A, Kinsella J. Inhibition of human LDL oxidation by resveratrol. Lancet. 1993; 341: 1103–1104.

Petroni A, Blasevich M, Salami M, Papini N, Montedoro GF, Galli C. Inhibition of platelet aggregation and eicosanoid production by phenolic components of olive oil. Thromb Res. 1995; 78: 151–160.

Pace-Asciak CR, Rounova O, Hahn SE, Diamandis EP, Goldberg DM. Wines and grape juices as modulators of platelet aggregation in healthy human subjects. Clin Chim Acta. 1996; 246: 163–182.

Martinez-Domingues E, de la Puerta R, Ruiz-Gutierrez V. Protective effects upon experimental inflammation models of a polyphenol-supplemented virgin olive oil diet. Inflamm Res. 2001; 50: 102–106.

Wallerath T, Deckert G, Ternes T, Anderson H, Li H, Witte K, Forstermann U. Resveratrol, a polyphenolic phytoalexin present in red wine, enhances expression and activity of endothelial nitric oxide synthase. Circulation. 2002; 106: 1652–1658.

Shan B, Cai YZ, Sun M, Corke H. Antioxidant capacity of 26 spice extracts and characterization of their phenolic constituents. J Agric Food Chem. 2005;53(20):7749–7759.

Jirovetz L, Buchbauer G, Stoilova I, Stoyanova A, Krastanov A, Schmidt E. Chemical composition and antioxidant properties of clove leaf essential oil. J Agric Food Chem. 2006;54(17):6303–6307.

Gülçin İ. Antioxidant activity of eugenol: a structure-activity relationship study. J Med Food. 2011;14(9):975–985.

Abdel-Wahhab MA, Aly SE. Antioxidant property of Nigella sativa (black cumin) and Syzygium aromaticum (clove) in rats during aflatoxicosis. J Appl Toxicol. 2005;25(3):218–223.

Halder S, Mehta AK, Kar R, Mustafa M, Mediratta PK, Sharma KK. Clove oil reverses learning and memory deficits in scopolamine-treated mice. Planta Med. 2011;77(8):830–834.

Rana IS, Rana AS, Rajak RC. Evaluation of antifungal activity in essential oil of the Syzygium aromaticum (L.) by extraction, purification and analysis of its main component eugenol. Braz J Microbiol. 2011;42(4):1269–1277.

Devi KP, Nisha SA, Sakthivel R, Pandian SK. Eugenol (an essential oil of clove) acts as an antibacterial agent against Salmonella typhi by disrupting the cellular membrane. J Ethnopharmacol. 2010;130(1):107–115.

Fu Y, Zu Y, Chen L, Shi X, Wang Z, Sun S, et al. et al. Antimicrobial activity of clove and rosemary essential oils alone and in combination. Phytother Res. 2007;21(10):989–994.

Ali SM, Khan AA, Ahmed I, Musaddiq M, Ahmed KS, Polasa H, et al. et al. Antimicrobial activities of eugenol and cinnamaldehyde against the human gastric pathogen Helicobacter pylori. Ann Clin Microbiol Antimicrob. 2005;4:20.

Hill LE, Gomes C, Taylor TM. Characterization of beta-cyclodextrin inclusion complexes containing essential oils (trans-cinnamaldehyde, eugenol, cinnamon bark, and clove bud extracts) for antimicrobial delivery applications. LWT-Food Sci Technol. 2013;51(1):86–93.

Daniel AN, Sartoretto SM, Schimidt G, Caparroz-Assef SM, Bersani-Amado CA, Cuman RK. Anti-inflamatory and antinociceptive activities of eugenol essential oil in experimental animal models. Rev Bras Farmacogn. 2009;19(1B):212–217.

Kurokawa M, Hozumi T, Basnet P, Nakano M, Kadota S, Namba T, et al. et al. Purification and characterization of eugeniin as an anti-herpesvirus compound from Geum japonicum and Syzygium aromaticum. J Pharmacol Exp Ther. 1998;284(2):728–735.

Ghosh R, Nadiminty N, Fitzpatrick JE, Alworth WL, Slaga TJ, Kumar AP. Eugenol causes melanoma growth suppression through inhibition of E2F1 transcriptional activity. J Biol Chem. 2005;280(7):5812–5819.

Gebhardt R, Beck H. Differential inhibitory effects of garlic-derived organosulfur compounds on cholesterol biosynthesis in primary rat hepatocyte cultures. Lipids. 1996;31(12):1269-1276.

Lawson LD, Ransom DK, Hughes BG. Inhibition of whole blood platelet-aggregation by compounds in garlic clove extracts and commercial garlic products. Thromb Res. 1992;65(2):141-156.

Dirsch VM, Kiemer AK, Wagner H, Vollmar AM. Effect of allicin and ajoene, two compounds of garlic, on inducible nitric oxide synthase. Atherosclerosis. 1998;139(2):333-339.

Chang HP, Huang SY, Chen YH. Modulation of cytokine secretion by garlic oil derivatives is associated with suppressed nitric oxide production in stimulated macrophages. J Agric Food Chem. 2005;53(7):2530-2534.

Keiss HP, Dirsch VM, Hartung T, et al. Garlic (*Allium sativum* L.) modulates cytokine expression in lipopolysaccharide-activated human blood thereby inhibiting NF-kappaB activity. J Nutr. 2003;133(7):2171-2175

Lefer DJ. A new gaseous signaling molecule emerges: cardioprotective role of hydrogen sulfide. Proc Natl Acad Sci U S A. 2007;104(46):17907-17908.

Munday R, Munday CM. Low doses of diallyl disulfide, a compound derived from garlic, increase tissue activities of quinone reductase and glutathione transferase in the gastrointestinal tract of the rat. Nutr Cancer. 1999;34(1):42-48.

Kweon S, Park KA, Choi H. Chemopreventive effect of garlic powder diet in diethylnitrosamine-induced rat hepatocarcinogenesis. Life Sci. 2003;73(19):2515-2526.

Stewart ZA, Westfall MD, Pietenpol JA. Cell-cycle dysregulation and anticancer therapy. Trends Pharmacol Sci. 2003;24(3):139-145.

Herman-Antosiewicz A, Singh SV. Signal transduction pathways leading to cell cycle arrest and apoptosis induction in cancer cells by *Allium* vegetable-derived organosulfur compounds: a review. Mutat Res. 2004;555(1-2):121-131.

Arunkumar A, Vijayababu MR, Srinivasan N, Aruldhas MM, Arunakaran J. Garlic compound, diallyl disulfide induces cell cycle arrest in prostate cancer cell line PC-3. Mol Cell Biochem. 2006;288(1-2):107-113.

Wu X, Kassie F, Mersch-Sundermann V. Induction of apoptosis in tumor cells by naturally occurring sulfur-containing compounds. Mutat Res. 2005;589(2):81-102.

Gail MH, Pfeiffer RM, Brown LM, et al. Garlic, vitamin, and antibiotic treatment for Helicobacter pylori: a randomized factorial controlled trial. Helicobacter. 2007;12(5):575-578.

Hu JF, Liu YY, Yu YK, Zhao TZ, Liu SD, Wang QQ. Diet and cancer of the colon and rectum: a case-control study in China. Int J Epidemiol. 1991;20(2):362-367.

Levi F, Pasche C, La Vecchia C, Lucchini F, Franceschi S. Food groups and colorectal cancer risk. Br J Cancer. 1999;79(7-8):1283-1287.

Giovannucci E, Rimm EB, Stampfer MJ, Colditz GA, Ascherio A, Willett WC. Intake of fat, meat, and fiber in relation to risk of colon cancer in men. Cancer Res. 1994;54(9):2390-2397.

Steinmetz KA, Kushi LH, Bostick RM, Folsom AR, Potter JD. Vegetables, fruit, and colon cancer in the Iowa Women's Health Study. Am J Epidemiol. 1994;139(1):1-15.

Chapter 4: References

Pisani P, Bray F, Parkin DM: Estimates of the world-wide prevalence of cancer for 25 sites in the adult population. Int J Cancer 97:72–81, 2002.

Pisani P, Parkin DM, Bray F, et al: Estimates of the worldwide mortality from 25 cancers in 1990. Int J Cancer 83:18–29, 1999.

Shimizu H, Ross RK, Bernstein L, et al: Cancers of the prostate and breast among Japanese and white immigrants in Los Angeles County. Br J Cancer 63:963–966, 1991.

Omenn GS, Goodman GE, Thornquist MD, et al: Risk factors for lung cancer and for intervention effects in CARET, the Beta-Carotene and Retinol

Efficacy Trial. J Natl Cancer Inst 88::1550, 1996–1559.

Stahl W, Nicolai S, Briviba K, et al: Biological activities of natural and synthetic carotenoids: Induction of gap junctional communication and singlet oxygen quenching. Carcinogenesis 18::89,1997–92.

Paganini-Hill A, Chao A, Ross RK, et al: Vitamin A, beta-carotene, and the risk of cancer: A prospective study. J Natl Cancer Inst 79::443,1987–448.

Campbell MJ, Koeffler HP: Toward therapeutic intervention of cancer by vitamin D compounds. J Natl Cancer Inst 89::182,1997–185.

Majeski S, Skopinska M, Marczak M, et al: Vitamin D is a potent inhibitor of tumor cell-induced angiogenesis. J Investig Dermatol Symp Proc 1::97,1996–101.

Blutt SE, McDonnell TJ, Polek TC, et al: Calcitriol-induced apoptosis in LNCaP cells is blocked by overexpression of bcl-2. Endocrinology 141::10,2000–17.

Albertsen PC, Fryback DG, Storer BE, et al: Long-term survival among men with conservatively treated localized prostate cancer. JAMA 274:626–631, 1995.

Wilkinson S, Gomella LG, Smith JA, et al: Attitudes and use of complementary therapy in men with prostate cancer. J Urol 168:2505–2509, 2002

Stivala LA, Savio M, Quarta S, et al: The antiproliferative effect of beta-carotene requires p21waf1/cip1 in normal human fibroblasts. Eur J Biochem 267:2290–2296, 2000.

Kotake-Nara E, Kushiro M, Zhang H, et al: Carotenoids affect proliferation of human prostate cancer cells. J Nutr 131:3303–3306, 2001.

Ribaya-Mercado JD, Holmgren SC, Fox JG, et al: Dietary beta-carotene absorption and metabolism in ferrets and rats. J Nutr 119:665–668, 1989

Hayes RB, Bogdanovicz JF, Schroeder FH, et al: Serum retinol and prostate cancer. Cancer 62:2021–2026, 1988

Ohno Y, Yoshida O, Oishi K, et al: Dietary beta-carotene and cancer of the prostate: A case-control study in Kyoto, Japan. Cancer Res 48:1331–1336, 1988.

Le Marchand L, Hankin JH, Kolonel LN, et al: Vegetable and fruit consumption in relation to prostate cancer risk in Hawaii: A reevaluation of the effect of dietary beta-carotene. Am J Epidemiol 133:215–219, 1991

Tzonou A, Signorello LB, Lagiou P, et al: Diet and cancer of the prostate: A case-control study in Greece. Int J Cancer 80:704–708, 1999.

Lu QY, Hung JC, Heber D, et al: Inverse associations between plasma lycopene and other carotenoids and prostate cancer. Cancer Epidemiol Biomarkers Prev 10:749–756, 2001.

Hsing AW, Comstock GW, Abbey H, et al: Serologic precursors of cancer: Retinol, carotenoids, and tocopherol and risk of prostate cancer. J Natl Cancer Inst 82:941–946, 1990.

Chapter 5: References

Almario RU, Vonghavaravat V, Wong R (2001). Effects of walnut consumption on plasma fatty acids and lipoproteins in combined hyperlipidemia. *Am J Clin Nutr.*; 74: 72 -79.

Bernacki, R. J., Niedbala, M. J. and Korytnyk, W. (1985) Glycosidases in cancer and invasion. Cancer Metastasis Rev. *4*, 81-102

Chen CY, Milbury PE, Lapsley K, Blumberg JB. (2005). Flavonoids from almond skins are bioavailable and act synergistically with vitamins C and E to enhance hamster and human LDL resistance to oxidation. J Nutr.;135:1366–73.

Dourado F, Barros A, Mota M, Coimbra MA, Gama FM. Anatomy and cell wall polysaccharides of almond (Prunus dulcis) seeds. J Agric Food Chem. 2004;52:1364–70.

Geetha T, Malhotra V, Chopra K, Kaur IP. (2005). Antimutagenic and antioxidant / prooxidant activity of quercetin. Indian J Exp Biol. Jan;43(1):61-7.

Hyson D, Schneeman B & Davis P (2002). Almonds and Almond Oil Have Similar Effects on Plasma Lipids and LDL Oxidation in Healthy Men and Women. J. Nutr., April 1, ; 132(4): 703 - 707.

Jaceldo-Siegl K, Sabate J, Rajaram S, Fraser GE. (2004). Long-term almond supplementation without advice on food replacement induces favourable nutrient modifications to the habitual diets of free-living individuals. Br J Nutr. Sep;92(3):533-40.

Jambazian PR, Haddad E, Rajaram S, Tanzman J, Sabate J. (2005). Almonds in the diet simultaneously improve plasma alpha-tocopherol concentrations and reduce plasma lipids. J Am Diet Assoc. Mar;105(3):449-54.

Jenkins D, Kendall C, Josse A, Salvatore S, Brighenti F, Augustin L, Ellis P, Vidgen E & Rao A (2006). Almonds Decrease Postprandial Glycemia, Insulinemia, and Oxidative Damage in Healthy Individuals. J Nutr. Dec;136(12):2987-2992.

Jenkins D, Kendall C, Marchie A. (2008). Almonds Reduce Biomarkers of Lipid Peroxidation in Older Hyperlipidemic Subjects. J Nutr; 138: 908-913

Kris-Etherton PM, Pearson TA, Wan Y, et al. (1999). High-monounsaturated fatty acid diets lower both plasma cholesterol and triglyceride concentrations. *Am J Clin Nutr.*; 70: 1009–1015.

Miller, A.A., M. Verghese, J. Boateng, L. Shackelford and L.T. Walker, (2010). Feeding almonds and pecans reduced development of azoxymethane-induced precancerous lesions. Int. J. Cancer Res., 6: 234-242.

Robinson, K. M., Begovic, M. E., Rhinehart, B. L., Heineke, E. W., Ducep, J.-B., Kastner, P. R., Marshall, F. N. and Danzin, C. (1991). New potent a-glucohydrolase inhibitor MDL 73945 with long duration of action in rats. Diabetes *40*, 825-830

Sang S, Lapsley K, Jeong WS, Lachance PA, Ho CT, Rosen RT. (2002). Antioxidative phenolic compounds isolated from almond skins (Prunus amygdalus Batsch). J Agric Food Chem.;50:2459–63.

Spiller GA, Jenkins DA, Bosello O, et al. (1998). Nuts and plasma lipids: an almond-based diet lowers LDL-C while preserving HDL-C. *J Am Coll Nutr.*; 17: 285–290.

Wien MA, Sabate JM, Ikle DN, Cole SE, Kandeel FR. (2003). Almonds vs complex carbohydrates in a weight reduction program. Int J Obes Relat Metab Disord. Nov 27(11):1365-72.

Chapter 6: References

Nahum A, Sharoni Y, Prall OW, Levy J, Hirsch K, Watts CK, Danilenko M (2001). "Lycopene inhibition of cell cycle progression in breast and endometrial cancer cells is associated with reduction in cyclin D levels and retention of p27(Kip1) in the cyclin E-cdk2 complexes". Oncogene 20 (26): 3428–436.

Karas M, Amir H, Fishman D, Danilenko M, Segal S, Nahum A, et al. Lycopene interferes with cell cycle progression and insulin-like growth factor I signaling in mammary cancer cells. Nutr Cancer 2000;36:101–11.

Chan JM, Stampfer MJ, Giovannucci E, Gann PH, Ma J, Wilkinson P, et al. Plasma insulin-like growth factor-I and prostate cancer risk: a prospective study. Science 1998;279:563–6.

Stattin P, Bylung A, Rinaldi S, Biessy C, Dechaud H, Stenman UH, et al. Plasma insulin-like growth factor-I, insulin-like growth factor-bind proteins, and prostate cancer risk: a prospective study. J Natl Cancer Inst 2000;92:1910–7.

Countryman C, Bankson D, Collins S, Mar B. Lycopene inhibits the growth of the HL-60 promyelocytic leukemia cell line. Clin Chem 1991;37:1056

Farinati F, Cardin R, Degan P, De Maria N, Floyd RA, Van Thiel DH.(1999). Oxidative DNA damage in circulating leukocytes occurs as an early event in chronic HCV infection. Free Radic Biol Med;27:1284–91.

Rao AV, Agarwal S.(1998). Bioavailability and in vivo antioxidant properties of lycopene from tomato products and their possible role in the prevention of cancer. Nutr Cancer;31:199–203.

Levy J, Sharoni Y, Danilenko M, Miinster A, Bosin E, Giat Y, Feldman B (1995). "Lycopene is a more potent inhibitor of human cancer cell proliferation than either alpha-carotene or beta-carotene". Nutr Cancer 24 (3): 257–266.

Narisawa T, Fukaura Y, Hasebe M, Ito M, Nishino H, Khachik F, Murakoshi M, Uemura S, Aizawa R (1996). "Ihibitory effects of natural carotenoids, alpha-carotene, beta-carotene, lycopene and lutein, on colonic aberrant crypt foci formation in rats.". Cancer Lett 107 (1): 137–142.

Wang, S., DeGroff, V. L. & Clinton, S. K. (2003) Tomato and soy polyphenols reduce insulin-like growth factor-1-stimulated rat prostate cancer cell proliferation and apoptotic resistance in vitro via inhibition of intracellular signaling pathways involving tyrosine kinase. J. Nutr. 133:2367-2376.

Chen, L., Stacewicz-Sapuntzakis, M., Duncan, C., Sharifi, R., Ghosh, L., van Breemen, R., Ashton, D. & Bowen, P. E. (2001) Oxidative DNA damage in prostate cancer patients consuming tomato sauce-based entrees as a whole-food intervention. J. Natl. Cancer Inst. 93:1872-1879.

Basu A, Imrhan V. (2007). Tomato versus lycopene in oxidative stress and carcinogenesis. Eur J Clin Nutr.;61(3):295-303..

Kucuk, O., Sarkar, F. H., Sakr, W., Djuric, Z., Pollak, M. N., Khachik, F., Li, Y. W., Banerjee, M. & Grignon, D., et al (2001) Phase II randomized clinical trial of lycopene supplementation before radical prostatectomy. Cancer Epidemiol. Biomarkers Prev. 10:861-868.

Beecher, G. R. (1998). Nutrient content of tomatoes and tomato products. Proc. Soc. Exp. Biol. Med. 218:98-100.

Tonucci, L., Holden, J., Beecher, G., Khackik, F., Davis, C. & Mulokozi, G. (1995) Carotenoid content of thermally processed tomato-based food products. J. Agric. Food Chem. 43:579-586.

Boileau, T. W., Liao, Z., Kim, S., Lemeshow, S., Erdman, J. W., Jr & Clinton, S. K. (2003) Prostate carcinogenesis in N-methyl-N-nitrosourea (NMU)-testosterone-treated rats fed tomato powder, lycopene, or energy-restricted diets. J. Natl. Cancer Inst. 95:1578-1586.

Rissanen, T., Voutilainen, S., Nyyssonen, K. & Salonon, J. (2002) Lycopene, atherosclerosis, and coronary heart disease. Exp. Biol. Med. 227:900-907.

Rissanen, T., Voutilainen, S., Nyyssonen, K., Salonon, J., Kaplan, G. & Salonen, J. (2003) Serum lycopene concentration and carotid atherosclerosis: the Kuopio Ischaemic Heart Disease Risk Factor Study. Am. J. Clin. Nutr. 77:133-138.

Kohlmeier, L., Kark, J. D., Gomez-Gracia, E., Martin, B. C., Steck, S. E., Kardinaal, A. F., Ringstad, J., Thamm, M. & Masaev, V., et al (1997) Lycopene and myocardial infarction risk in the EURAMIC Study. Am. J. Epidemiol. 146:618-626.

Sesso, H. D., Liu, S., Gaziano, J. M. & Buring, J. E. (2003) Dietary lycopene, tomato-based food products and cardiovascular disease in women. J. Nutr. 133:2336-2341.

Sesso, H. D., Buring, J. E., Norkus, E. P. & Gaziano, J. M. (2004) Plasma lycopene, other carotenoids, and retinol and the risk of cardiovascular disease in women. Am. J. Clin. Nutr. 79:47-53.

Di Mascio P, Kaiser S, Sies H (1989). "Lycopene as the most efficient biological carotenoid singlet oxygen quencher". Arch. Biochem. Biophys. 274 (2): 532–8.

Gerster H (1997). "The potential role of lycopene for human health". J Am Coll Nutr 16 (2): 109–26.

Stewart, A., Bozonnet, S., Mullen, W., Jenkins, G., Lean, M. & Crozier, A. (2000) Occurrence of flavonols in tomatoes and tomato-based products. J. Agric. Food Chem. 48:2663-2669.

USDA National Nutrient Database for Standard Reference, Release 16–1 2004 Lycopene Content of Selected Foods, Per Common Measure, Sorted by Nutrient Content.

Gann, P., Ma, J., Giovannucci, E., Willett, W., Sacks, F., Hennekens, C. & Stampfer, M. (1999) Lower prostate cancer risk in men with elevated plasma lycopene levels: results of a prospective analysis. Cancer Res. 59:1225-1230.

Lu, Q., Hung, J., Heber, D., Go, V., Reuter, V., Crordon-Cardo, C., Scher, H., Marshall, J. & Zhang, Z. (2001) Inverse associations between plasma lycopene and other carotenoids and prostate cancer. Cancer Epidemiol. Biomarkers Prev. 10:749-756.

Giovannucci, E., Rimm, E., Liu, Y., Stampfer, M. & Willett, W. (2002) A prospective study of tomato products, lycopene, and prostate cancer risk. J. Natl. Cancer Inst. 94:391-398.

Etminan, M., Takkouche, B. & Caamano-Asorna, F. (2004) The role of tomato products and lycopene in the prevention of prostate cancer: a meta-analysis of observational studies. Cancer Epidemiol. Biomarkers Prev. 13:340-345.

Ellinger S, Ellinger J, Stehle P. (2006) Tomatoes, tomato products and lycopene in the prevention and treatment of prostate cancer: do we have the evidence from intervention studies? Curr Opin Clin Nutr Metab Care. 9(6):722-7.

Chapter 7 & 8: Oxidative Stress References

Barber MD, Powell JJ, Lynch SF, Fearon KC, and Ross JA. A polymorphism of the interleukin-1 β gene influences survival in pancreatic cancer. *Br J Cancer* 83: 1443-1447, 2000.

Barbera-Guillem E, Nyhus JK, Wolford CC, Friece CR, and Sampsel JW. Vascular endothelial growth factor secretion by tumor-infiltrating macrophages essentially supports tumor angiogenesis, and IgG immune complexes potentiate the process. *Cancer Res* 62: 7042-7049, 2002.

Bromberg J and Darnell Jr. JE The role of STATs in transcriptional control and their impact on cellular function. *Oncogene* 19: 2468-2473, 2000.

Cotran RS, Kumar V, and Collins T. *Pathologic Basis of Disease*. Philadelphia: Saunders, 1999.

Coussens LM and Werb Z. Inflammation and cancer. *Nature* 420: 860-867, 2002.

Cramer T, Yamanishi Y, Clausen BE, Forster I, Pawlinski R, Mackman N, Haase VH, Jaenisch R, Corr M, Nizet V, Firestein GS, Gerber HP, Ferrara N, and Johnson RS. HIF-1α is essential for myeloid cell-mediated inflammation. *Cell* 112: 645-657, 2003.

Dalgleish AG and O'Byrne KJ. Chronic immune activation and inflammation in the pathogenesis of AIDS and cancer. *Adv Cancer Res* 84: 231-276, 2002.

De Jong MM, Nolte IM, te Meerman GJ, van der Graaf WT, de Vries EG, Sijmons RH, Hofstra RM, and Kleibeuker JH. Low-penetrance genes and their involvement in colorectal cancer susceptibility. *Cancer Epidemiol Biomarkers Prev* 11: 1332-1352, 2002.

El-Omar EM. The importance of interleukin 1β in *Helicobacter pylori* associated disease. *Gut* 48: 743-747, 2001.

El-Omar EM, Carrington M, Chow WH, McColl KE, Bream JH, Young HA, Herrera J, Lissowska J, Yuan CC, Rothman N, Lanyon G, Martin M, Fraumeni JF Jr, and Rabkin CS. Interleukin-1 polymorphisms associated with increased risk of gastric cancer. *Nature* 404: 398-402, 2000.

Gupta RA, Polk DB, Krishna U, Israel DA, Yan F, DuBois RN, and Peek RM Jr. Activation of peroxisome proliferator-activated receptor gamma suppresses nuclear factor κB-mediated apoptosis induced by *Helicobacter pylori* in gastric epithelial cells. *J Biol Chem* 276: 31059-31066, 2001.

Jackson PA, Green MA, Marks CG, King RJ, Hubbard R, and Cook MG. Lymphocyte subset infiltration patterns and HLA antigen status in colorectal carcinomas and adenomas. *Gut* 38: 85-89, 1996.

Jaiswal M, LaRusso NF, and Gores GJ. Nitric oxide in gastrointestinal epithelial cell carcinogenesis: linking inflammation to oncogenesis. *Am J Physiol Gastrointest Liver Physiol* 281: G626-G634, 2001.

Chapter 9: References

Breathnach AS (1999). Azelaic acid: potential as a general antitumoural agent. Med Hypotheses. 52(3):221-6.

Nazzaro-Porro, M, Passi, S, Balus, L, Breathnach, AS: Effect of dicarboxylic acids. J Invest Dermatol 1979 72: 296–305.

Manosroi A, Panyosak A, Rojanasakul Y, Manosroi J. (2007). Characteristics and antiproliferative activity of azelaic acid and its derivatives entrapped in bilayer vesicles in cancer cell lines. J Drug Target. 15(5):334-41.

Pathak, MA, Farinelli, WA, Fitzpatrick, TB: Cutaneous depigmentation by certain antioxidants, azelaic acid and DOPA derivatives. Clin Res 1979 27: 244A,

Ward, BJ, Breathnach, AS, Robins, EJ, Bhasin, Y, Ethridge, L, Passi, S, Nazzarro-Porro, M: Analytical, ultrastructural, autoradiographic and biochemical studies on (^{3}H) dicarboxylic acid added to cultures of melanoma cells. Br J Dermatol 1984 111: 29–36.

Laemmli, UK: Cleavage of structural proteins during the assembly of the head of bacteriophage T4. Nature 1970 227: 680–685.

Spona, J, Leibl, H: Inhibition by tamoxifen of estrogen stimulated accumulation of preprolactin messenger ribonucleic acid. Biochim Biophys Acta 1981 656: 45–54.

Nazzaro-Porro, M, Passi, S, Zina, G, Bernengo, A, Breathnach, A, Gallagher, S, Morpurgo, G: Effect of azelaic acid on human malignant melanoma. Lancet 1980 1: 1109–1111.

Lotan, R, Neumann, G, Lotan, D: Relationship among retinoid structure, inhibition of growth and cellular retinoic acid-binding protein in cultured S 91 melanoma cells. Cancer Res 1980 40: 1097–1102.

Fischer MJ, Paulussen JJ, Horbach DA, Roelofsen EP, van Miltenburg JC, de Mol NJ, Janssen LH. (1995). Inhibition of mediator release in RBL-2H3 cells by some H1-antagonist derived anti-allergic drugs: relation to lipophilicity and membrane effects. Inflamm Res. Feb;44(2):92-7.

Adams W, Morris D L. Short-course cimetidine and survival with colorectal cancer. Lancet 1994; 344: 1768-9.

Adams W J, Morris D L. Pilot study cimetidine enhances lymphocyte infiltration of human colorectal carcinoma: results of a small randomized control trial. Cancer 1997; 80: 15-21.

Armitage J O, Sidner R D. Antitumour effect of cimetidine? Lancet 1979; i: 882-3.

Borgström S, et al. Human leukocyte interferon and cimetidine for metastatic melanoma. N Eng J Med 1982; 307: 1080-81.

Gifford R R M, Fergusson R M, Voss B V. (1981). Cimetidine reduction of tumour formation in mice. Lancet; i: 638-40.

Hahm K B, et al. Comparison of antiproliferative effects of 1-histamine-2 receptor antagonists, cimetidine, ranitidine, and famotidine, in gastric cancer cells. Int J Immunopharmacol . (1996); 18: 393-9

Lawson J A, Adams W, Morris D L. Ranitidine and cimetidine differ in their in vitro and in vivo effects on human colonic cancer growth. Br J Cancer. (1996). 73: 872-6.

Matsumoto S. Cimetidine and survival with colorectal cancer. Lancet (1995); 346: 115.

Thornes R D, Lynch G. Combination of cimetidine with other drugs for treatment of cancer. N Eng J Med 1983; 308: 591.

Takahashi HK, Watanabe T, Yokoyama A, Iwagaki H, Yoshino T, Tanaka N, Nishibori M. (2006) Cimetidine induces interleukin-18 production through H2-agonist activity in monocytes. Mol Pharmacol. 70(2):450-3.

Fukuda M, Kusama K, Sakashita H. (2008). Cimetidine inhibits salivary gland tumor cell adhesion to neural cells and induces apoptosis by blocking NCAM expression. BMC Cancer. 18;8:376

Kubecova M, Kolostova K, Pinterova D, Kacprzak G, Bobek V. (2011). Cimetidine: an anticancer drug? Eur J Pharm Sci. 42(5):439-44.

Eichbaum C, Meyer AS, Wang N, Bischofs E, Steinborn A, Bruckner T, Brodt P, Sohn C, Eichbaum MH. (2011). Breast cancer cell-derived cytokines, macrophages and cell adhesion: implications for metastasis. Anticancer Res. (10):3219-27

Baur M, van Oosterom AT, Diéras V, Tubiana-Hulin M, Coombes RC, Hatschek T, Murawsky M, Klink-Alakl M, Hudec M. (2008) A phase II trial of docetaxel (Taxotere) as second-line chemotherapy in patients with metastatic breast cancer. J Cancer Res Clin Oncol. 134(2):125-35.

Ben-Chetrit E, Amir G, Shalit M (February 2005). "Cetirizine: An effective agent in Kimura's disease". Arthritis Rheum. 53 (1): 117–8.

Jankowska H, Hooper P, Jankowski JA. (2010)Aspirin chemoprevention of gastrointestinal cancer in the next decade. A review of the evidence. Pol Arch Med Wewn. 120(10):407-12.

Chen JW, Zhou SB, Tan ZM. (2010). Aspirin and pravastatin reduce lectin-like oxidized low density lipoprotein receptor-1 expression, adhesion molecules and oxidative stress in human coronary artery endothelial cells. Chin Med J (Engl). 123(12):1553-6.

Yusuf SW, Iliescu C, Bathina JD, Daher IN, Durand JB. (2010). Antiplatelet therapy and percutaneous coronary intervention in patients with acute coronary syndrome and thrombocytopenia. Tex Heart Inst J.;37(3):336-40.

Ghosh N, Chaki R, Mandal V, Mandal SC. (2010). COX-2 as a target for cancer chemotherapy. Pharmacol Rep. 62(2):233-44.

Cronin-Fenton DP, Pedersen L, Lash TL, Friis S, Baron JA, Sørensen HT. (2010). Prescriptions for selective cyclooxygenase-2 inhibitors, non-selective non-steroidal anti-inflammatory drugs, and risk of breast cancer in a population-based case-control study. Breast Cancer Res.;12(2):R15.

Asgari MM, Chren MM, Warton EM, Friedman GD, White E. (2010). Association between nonsteroidal anti-inflammatory drug use and cutaneous squamous cell carcinoma. Arch Dermatol.;146(4):388-95.

Bodelon C, Doherty JA, Chen C, Rossing MA, Weiss NS. 2009). Use of nonsteroidal anti-inflammatory drugs and risk of endometrial cancer. Am J Epidemiol. 170(12):1512-7.

Thun MJ, Henley SJ, Patrono C*(2002)*. *Nonsteroidal anti-inflammatory drugs as anticancer agents: mechanistic, pharmacologic, and clinical issues. J Natl Cancer Inst;94:252-66.*

Wang D, Dubois RN. *(2006). Prostaglandins and cancer. Gut;55:115-22.*

Baron JA, Cole BF, Sandler RS, Haile RW, Ahnen D, Bresalier R, *(2003). A randomized trial of aspirin to prevent colorectal adenomas. N Engl J Med;348:891-9.*

Sandler RS, Halabi S, Baron JA, Budinger S, Paskett E, Keresztes R, *(2003). A randomized trial of aspirin to prevent colorectal adenomas in patients with previous colorectal cancer. N Engl J Med;348:883-90.*

Gonzalez-Perez A, Rodriguez LAG, Lopez-Ridaura R. *(2003). Effects of non-steroidal anti-inflammatory drugs on cancer sites other than the colon and rectum: a meta-analysis. BMC Cancer;3:28.*

Mahmud S, Franco E, Aprikian A *(2004). Prostate cancer and use of nonsteroidal anti-inflammatory drugs: systematic review and meta-analysis. Br J Cancer;90:93-9.*

Khuder SA, Herial NA, Mutgi AB, Federman DJ. *(2005). Nonsteroidal antiinflammatory drug use and lung cancer: a metaanalysis. Chest;127:748-54.*

Shekelle P, Hardy ML, Coulter I, Udani J, Spar M, Oda K. Effect of the supplemental use of antioxidants vitamin C, vitamin E, and coenzyme Q10 for the prevention and treatment of cancer. *Evid Rep Technol Assess (Summ)* 2003;75:1–3.

Hertz N, Lister RE. (2009) Improved survival in patients with end-stage cancer treated with coenzyme Q(10) and other antioxidants: a pilot study. J Int Med Res. Nov-Dec;37(6):1961-71.

Yuvaraj S, Premkumar VG, Shanthi P, Vijayasarathy K, Gangadaran SG, Sachdanandam P. (2009). Effect of Coenzyme Q(10), Riboflavin and Niacin on Tamoxifen treated postmenopausal breast cancer women with special reference to blood chemistry profiles. Breast Cancer Res Treat. Mar;114(2):377-84.

Nohl H, Gille L, Kozlov AV (1999) Critical aspects of the antioxidant function of coenzyme Q in biomembranes. Biofactors 9:155- 161

Al-Hasso. Coenzyme Q10: a review. *Hosp Pharm.* (2001);36(1):51-66.

Beal MF. Therapeutic effects of coenzyme Q10 in neurodegenerative diseases. *Methods Enzymol.* (2004) ;382:473-87.

Belardinelli R, Mucaj A, Lacalaprice F, et al., Coenzyme Q10 and exercise training in chronic heart failure. *Eur Heart J.* 2006;27(22):2675-81.

Caso G, Kelly P, McNurlan MA, Lawson WE. Effect of coenzyme q10 on myopathyic symptoms in patients treated with statins. *Am J Cardiol.* (2007);99(10):1409-12.

Dhanasekaran M, Ren J. The emerging role of coenzyme Q-10 in aging, neurodegeneration, cardiovascular disease, cancer and diabetes mellitus. *Curr Neurovasc Res.* (2005);2(5):447-59.

Villalba JM, Parrado C, Santos-Gonzalez M, Alcain FJ . (2010) Therapeutic use of coenzyme Q10 and coenzyme Q10-related compounds and formulations. Expert Opin Investig Drugs. Apr;19(4):535-54.

Lockwood K., Moesgaard S., Yamamoto T. and Folkers K. (1995). Progress on Therapy of Breast Cancer with Vitamin Q_{10} and the Regression of Metastases. Biochemical and Biophysical Research Communication. Volume 212, Issue 1, 172-177

Yuvaraj S, Premkumar VG, Vijayasarathy K, Gangadaran SG, Sachdanandam P. Ameliorating effect of coenzyme Q10, riboflavin and niacin in tamoxifen-treated postmenopausal breast cancer patients with special reference to lipids and lipoproteins. *Clin Biochem. (2007)*;40:623–8.

Adhikary A, Mohanty S, Lahiry L, Hossain DM, Chakraborty S, Das T. Theaflavins retard human breast cancer cell migration by inhibiting NF-kappaB via p53-ROS cross-talk. *FEBS Lett.* 2010;584:7–14.

Chao HP, Kuo CD, Chiu JH, Fu SL. Andrographolide Exhibits Anti-Invasive Activity against Colon Cancer Cells via Inhibition of MMP2 Activity. *Planta Med.* 2010.

Littarru GP, Tiano L. Clinical aspects of coenzyme Q10: an update. *Nutrition.* 2010;26:250–4.

Portakal O, Ozkaya O, Erden Inal M, Bozan B, Kosan M, Sayek I. coenzyme Q10 concentrations and antioxidant status in tissues of breast cancer patients. *Clin Biochem.* 2000;33:279–284.

Hertz N, Lister RE. Improved survival in patients with end-stage cancer treated with coenzyme Q(10) and other antioxidants: a pilot study. *J Int Med Res.* 2010;38:293.

Sachdanandam P. Antiangiogenic and hypolipidemic activity of coenzyme Q10 supplementation to breast cancer patients undergoing Tamoxifen therapy. *Biofactors.* 2008;32:151–9.

Premkumar VG, Yuvaraj S, Vijayasarathy K, Gangadaran SG, Sachdanandam P. Effect of coenzyme Q10, riboflavin and niacin on serum CEA and CA 15-3 levels in breast cancer patients undergoing tamoxifen therapy. *Biol Pharm Bull.* 2007;30:367–70.

Premkumar VG, Yuvaraj S, Sathish S, Shanthi P, Sachdanandam P. Anti-angiogenic potential of CoenzymeQ10, riboflavin and niacin in breast cancer patients undergoing tamoxifen therapy. *Vascul Pharmacol.* 2008;48:191–201.

Rusciani L, Proietti I, Rusciani A, Paradisi A, Sbordoni G, Alfano C. Low plasma coenzyme Q10 levels as an independent prognostic factor for melanoma progression. *J Am Acad Dermatol.* 2006;**54**:234–41.

Ho YS, Lai CS, Liu HI, Ho SY, Tai C, Pan MH, Wang YJ. Dihydrolipoic acid inhibits skin tumor promotion through anti-inflammation and anti-oxidation. *Biochem Pharmacol.* 2007;**73**:1786–1795.

Selvakumar E, Hsieh TC. 2008. Regulation of cell cycle transition and induction of apoptosis in HL-60 leukemia cells by lipoic acid: role in cancer prevention and therapy. *J Hematol Oncol.* May 30;1:4.

Rao PK. Efficacy of alpha lipoic acid in adjunct with intralesional steroids and hyaluronidase in the management of oral submucous fibrosis. *J Cancer Res Ther.* 2010 Oct-Dec;6(4):508-10.

Bhavsar SK, Bobbala D, Xuan NT, Föller M, Lang F. Stimulation of suicidal erythrocyte death by α-lipoic acid. *Cell Physiol Biochem.* 2010;26(6):859-68.

Gianturco V, Bellomo A, D'ottavio E, Formosa V, Iori A, Mancinella M, Troisi G, Marigliano V (2009). "Impact of therapy with alpha-lipoic acid (ALA) on the oxidative stress in the controlled NIDDM: a possible preventive way against the organ dysfunction?". *Archives of gerontology and geriatrics* 49 Suppl 1: 129–33.

Morcos M, Borcea V, Isermann B, Gehrke S, Ehret T, Henkels M, Schiekofer S, Hofmann M et al. (June 2001). "Effect of alpha-lipoic acid on the progression of endothelial cell damage and albuminuria in patients with diabetes mellitus: an exploratory study". *Diabetes research and clinical practice* 52 (3): 175–83.

Ghibu S, Richard C, Vergely C, Zeller M, Cottin Y, Rochette L (November 2009). "Antioxidant properties of an endogenous thiol: Alpha-lipoic acid, useful in the prevention of cardiovascular diseases". *Journal of cardiovascular pharmacology* 54 (5): 391–8.

Alleva R, Nasole E, Di Donato F, Borghi B, Neuzil J, Tomasetti M (July 2005). "alpha-Lipoic acid supplementation inhibits oxidative damage, accelerating chronic wound healing in patients undergoing hyperbaric oxygen therapy". *Biochemical and biophysical research communications* 333 (2): 404–10.

Chang JW, Lee EK, Kim TH, Min WK, Chun S, Lee KU, Kim SB, Park JS (2007). "Effects of alpha-lipoic acid on the plasma levels of asymmetric dimethylarginine in diabetic end-stage renal disease patients on hemodialysis: a pilot study". *American journal of nephrology* **27** (1): 70–4.

Ying Z, Kherada N, Farrar B, Kampfrath T, Chung Y, Simonetti O, Deiuliis J, Desikan R et al. (2010). "Lipoic acid effects on established atherosclerosis". *Life sciences* 86 (3–4): 95–102.

Garcion, E; Wionbarbot, N; Monteromenei, C; Berger, F; Wion, D (2002). "New clues about vitamin D functions in the nervous system". *Trends in Endocrinology and Metabolism* **13** (3): 100–5.

Kim KN, Pie JE, Park JH, Park YH, Kim HW, Kim MK. Retinoic acid and ascorbic acid act synergistically in inhibiting human breast cancer cell proliferation. J Nutr Biochem. 2006 Jul;17(7):454-62

Larsson SC, Bergkvist L, Näslund I, Rutegård J, Wolk A. Vitamin A, retinol, and carotenoids and the risk of gastric cancer: a prospective cohort study. Am J Clin Nutr. 2007 Feb;85(2):497-503.

Chan LN, Zhang S, Shao J, Waikel R, Thompson EA, Chan TS. N-(4-hydroxyphenyl)retinamide induces apoptosis in T lymphoma and T lymphoblastoid leukemia cells. Leuk Lymphoma. 1997 Apr;25(3-4):271-80.

Balendiran, Ganesaratnam K.; Dabur, Rajesh; Fraser, Deborah (2004). "The role of glutathione in cancer". *Cell Biochemistry and Function* **22** (6): 343–52

Escárcega RO, Fuentes-Alexandro S, García-Carrasco M, Gatica A, Zamora A (2007). "The transcription factor nuclear factor-κB and cancer". *Clinical Oncology (Royal College of Radiologists (Great Britain))* **19** (2): 154–61.

Paur I, Balstad TR, Kolberg M, Pedersen MK, Austenaa LM, Jacobs DR, Blomhoff R (May 2010). "Extract of oregano, coffee, thyme, clove, and walnuts inhibits NF-kappaB in monocytes and in transgenic reporter mice". *Cancer Prev Res (Phila)* **3** (5): 653–63.

Kohen R & Nyska A. (2002) Oxidation of Biological Systems: Oxidative Stress

Phenomena, Antioxidants, Redox Reactions, and Methods for Their Quantification Toxicol Pathol vol. 30, no. 6, 620-650.

Conn, P. F., Schalch, W. & Truscott, T. G. (1991) The singlet oxygen and carotenoid interaction. J. Photochem. Photobiol. B 11:41-47.

Nelsom, W. G., De Marzo, A. M. & Isaacs, W. B. (2003) Mechanisms of disease: prostate cancer. N. Engl. J. Med. 349:366-381.

Ames BN. Dietary carcinogens and anticarcinogens. Oxygen radicals and degenerative diseases. Science 1983;221:1256–64.

Guyton KZ, Kensler TW. Oxidative mechanisms in carcinogenesis. Br Med Bull 1993;49:523–44.

Law, N.; Caudle, M; Pecoraro, V (1998). *Manganese Redox Enzymes and Model Systems: Properties, Structures, and Reactivity.* 46. p. 305.

Herrera; Barbas, C (2001). "Vitamin E: action, metabolism and perspectives". *Journal of physiology and biochemistry* 57 (2): 43–56.

Packer L, Weber SU, Rimbach G; Traber (February 2001). "MoB journal : official publication of the Federation of American Societies for Experimental Biology". *Journal of Nutrition* 131 (2): 369S–73S.

Wefers, H; Sics (1988). "The protection of ascorbate and glutathione against microsomal lipid peroxidation is dependent on Vitamin E". *European Journal of Biochemistry* 174 (2): 353–357.

Ruano-Ravina A, Figueiras A, Freire-Garabal M, Barros-Dios JM (2006). "Antioxidant vitamins and risk of lung cancer". *Curr. Pharm. Des.* 12 (5): 599–613

Freeland-Graves J, Llanes C. Models to study manganese deficiency. In: Klimis-Tavantzis DL, ed. Manganese in health and disease. Boca Raton: CRC Press, Inc; 1994.

Odabasi E, Turan M, Aydin A, Akay C, Kutlu M. Magnesium, zinc, copper, manganese, and selenium levels in postmenopausal women with osteoporosis. Can magnesium play a key role in osteoporosis? Ann Acad Med Singapore. 2008;37(7):564-567.

Carl GF, Gallagher BB. Manganese and epilepsy. In: Klimis-Tavantzis DL, ed. Manganese in health and disease. Boca Raton: CRC Press, Inc; 1994:133-157.

Nilsonne G, Sun X, Nyström C, *et al.* (2006). "Selenite induces apoptosis in sarcomatoid malignant mesothelioma cells through oxidative stress". *Free Radical Biology & Medicine* 41 (6): 874–85.

Tsavachidou D, McDonnell TJ, Wen S, *et al.* (2009). "Selenium and vitamin E: cell type- and intervention-specific tissue effects in prostate cancer". *Journal of the National Cancer Institute* 101 (5): 306–20.

Zeng, H. and Combs, G. F. Jr. (2007). Selenium as an anticancer nutrient: roles in cell proliferation and tumor cell invasion. *J. Nutr. Biochem.* 19, 1-7.

Pool-Zobel, B. L., Bub, A., Muller, H., Wollowski, I. & Rechkemmer, G. (1997) Consumption of vegetables reduces genetic damage in humans: first results of a human intervention trial with carotenoid-rich foods. Carcinogenesis 18:1847-1850.

Russel, R.M. (2002). Beta-carotene and lung cancer. *Pure Appl. Chem.* 74 (8): 1461–1467.

Tanvetyanon T, Bepler G (July 2008). "Beta-carotene in multivitamins and the possible risk of lung cancer among smokers versus former smokers: a meta-analysis and evaluation of national brands". *Cancer* 113 (1): 150–7.

Zhang CX, Ho SC, Chen YM, Fu JH, Cheng SZ, Lin FY (2009). "Greater vegetable and fruit intake is associated with a lower risk of breast cancer among Chinese women". *International Journal of Cancer* 125 (1): 181–8.

Freedman ND, Park Y, Subar AF, *et al.* (May 2008). "Fruit and vegetable intake and head and neck cancer risk in a large United States prospective cohort study". *International Journal of Cancer* 122 (10): 2330–6.

Armstrong GA, Hearst JE (1996). "Carotenoids 2: Genetics and molecular biology of carotenoid pigment biosynthesis". *FASEB J.* 10 (2): 228–37.

Giovannucci E, Ascherio A, Rimm EB, Stampfer MJ, Colditz GA, Willett WC (1995). "Intake of carotenoids and retinol in relation to risk of prostate cancer". *J. Natl. Cancer Inst.* 87 (23): 1767–76.

Grossman AR, Lohr M, Im CS (2004). "Chlamydomonas reinhardtii in the landscape of pigments". *Annu. Rev. Genet.* 38: 119–73.

IARC Working Group on the Evaluation of Cancer Preventive Agents (1998). *IARC Handbooks of Cancer Prevention: Volume 2: Carotenoids (IARC Handbooks of Cancer Prevention)*. Oxford University Press, USA. pp. 25.

Khan N, Afaq F, Mukhtar H (2008). "Cancer chemoprevention through dietary antioxidants: progress and promise". *Antioxid. Redox Signal.* **10** (3): 475–510.

Rao AV, Balachandran B (2002). "Role of oxidative stress and antioxidants in neurodegenerative diseases". *Nutritional Neuroscience* **5** (5): 291–309

Rao AV, Rao LG (March 2007). "Carotenoids and human health". *Pharmacol. Res.* **55** (3): 207–16.

Harman, D (1956). "Aging: a theory based on free radical and radiation chemistry". Journal of Gerontology 11 (3): 298-300.

Harman, D (1972). "A biologic clock: the mitochondria?". Journal of the American Geriatrics Society 20 (4): 145-147.

Ishii N (2000). "Oxidative stress and aging in Caenorhabditis elegans". Free Radical Research 33 (6): 857-64.

Larsen P (1993). "<u>Aging and resistance to oxidative damage in Caenorhabditis elegans</u>". Proc Natl Acad Sci U S A 90 (19): 8905-9.

Sohal R, Mockett R, Orr W (2002). "Mechanisms of aging: an appraisal of the oxidative stress hypothesis". Free Radic Biol Med 33 (5): 575-86.

Rattan S (2006).Theories of biological aging: genes, proteins, and free radicals. Free Radic Res 40 (12): 1230-8

Mattson MP (2005). "Energy intake, meal frequency, and health: a neurobiological perspective.". Annual Review of Nutrition 25 (25): 237-60.

Muller, F. L., Lustgarten, M. S., Jang, Y., Richardson, A. and Van Remmen, H. (2007). "Trends in oxidative aging theories". Free Radical Biology & Medicine 43 (4): 477-503.

de Diego-Otero Y, Romero-Zerbo Y, el Bekay R, Decara J, Sanchez L, Rodriguez-de Fonseca F, del Arco-Herrera I. (March 2009). "Alpha-tocopherol protects against oxidative stress in the fragile X knockout mouse: an experimental therapeutic approach for the Fmr1 deficiency.". Neuropsychopharmacology 34 (4): 1011–26.

Gems D, Partridge L (March 2008). "Stress-response hormesis and aging: "that which does not kill us makes us stronger"". Cell Metab. 7 (3): 200–3.

Schafer FQ, Buettner GR (2001). "Redox environment of the cell as viewed through the redox state of the glutathione disulfide/glutathione couple". Free Radic. Biol. Med. 30 (11): 1191–212.

Lennon SV, Martin SJ, Cotter TG (1991). "Dose-dependent induction of apoptosis in human tumour cell lines by widely diverging stimuli". Cell Prolif. 24 (2): 203–14.

Valko M, Morris H, Cronin MT (May 2005). "Metals, toxicity and oxidative stress". Curr. Med. Chem. 12 (10): 1161–208.

Evans MD, Cooke MS. Factors contributing to the outcome of oxidative damage to nucleic acids. Bioessays. 2004 May;26(5):533–42.

Lee YJ, Shacter E (1999). "Oxidative stress inhibits apoptosis in human lymphoma cells". J. Biol. Chem. 274 (28): 19792–8.

Messner KR, Imlay JA (November 2002). "Mechanism of superoxide and hydrogen peroxide formation by fumarate reductase, succinate dehydrogenase, and aspartate oxidase". J. Biol. Chem. 277 (45): 42563–71.

Meyers DG, Maloley PA, Weeks D (1996). "Safety of antioxidant vitamins". Arch. Intern. Med. 156 (9): 925–35.

Ruano-Ravina A, Figueiras A, Freire-Garabal M, Barros-Dios JM (2006). "Antioxidant vitamins and risk of lung cancer". Curr. Pharm. Des. 12 (5): 599–613.

Pryor WA (2000). "Vitamin E and heart disease: basic science to clinical intervention trials". Free Radic. Biol. Med. 28 (1): 141–64.

Boothby LA, Doering PL (2005). "Vitamin C and vitamin E for Alzheimer's disease". Ann Pharmacother 39 (12): 2073–80.

Kontush K, Schekatolina S (2004). "Vitamin E in neurodegenerative disorders: Alzheimer's disease". Ann. N. Y. Acad. Sci. 1031: 249–62.

Nathan C, Shiloh MU (2000). "Reactive oxygen and nitrogen intermediates in the relationship between mammalian hosts and microbial pathogens". Proc. Natl. Acad. Sci. U.S.A. 97 (16): 8841–8.

Portugal-Cohen Meital; Numa Ran; Yaka Rami; Kohen Ron (2010). Cocaine induces oxidative damage to skin via xanthine oxidase and nitric oxide synthase. Journal of dermatological science 2010;58(2):105-12.

Rebecca Chinery, R. Daniel Beauchamp, Yu Shyr, Susan C. Kirkland, Robert J. Coffey, & Jason D. Morrow (1998). Antioxidants reduce cyclooxygenase-2 expression, prostaglandin production, and proliferation in colorectal cancer cells. Cancer Res June 1, *58;* 2323.

Ian D. Coulter, Mary L. Hardy, Sally C. Morton, Lara G. Hilton[1], Wenli Tu, Di Valentine, Paul G. Shekelle (2006). Antioxidants vitamin C and vitamin e for the prevention and treatment of cancer. Journal of General Internal Medicine. Vol 21,7, 735-744,

Deepak P Vivekananthan, Marc S Penn, Shelly K Sapp, Amy Hsu, Eric J Topol (2003) Use of antioxidant vitamins for the prevention of cardiovascular disease: meta-analysis of randomised trials The Lancet, Volume 361, Issue 9374, Pages 2017 - 2023,

Chapter 10: References

Andersen, B.L., Farrar, W.B., Golden-Kreutz, D., Kutz, L.A., MacCallum, R., Courtney, M.E., et al. (1998). Stress and immune responses after surgical treatment for regional breast cancer. Journal of the National Cancer Institute, 90, 30–36.

Andrews G: Placebo response in depression: bane of research, boon to therapy. Br J Psychiatry 2001; 178:192-194.

Bench CJ, Frackowiak RSJ, Dolan RJ: Changes in regional cerebral blood flow on recovery from depression. Psychol Med 1995; 25:247-251

Buckingham, J.C., Giles, G.E., & Cowell, A. (1997). Stress, stress hormones, and the immune system. Chichester, UK: Wiley.

Cohen, F., Kearney, K.A., Zegans, L.S., Kemeny, M.E., Neuhaus, J.M., & Stites, D.P. (1999). Differential immune system changes with acute and persistent stress for optimists vs pessimists. Brain Behavior and Immunity, **13**, 155–174.

Enserink M: Can the placebo be the cure? Science 1999; 284:238-240.

Hrobjartsson A, Gotzsche PC: Is the placebo powerless? an analysis of clinical trials comparing placebo with no treatment. N Engl J Med 2001; 344:1594-

Jensen MP, Karoly P: Motivation and expectancy factors in symptoms perception: a laboratory study of the placebo effect. Psychosom Med 1991; 53:144-152

Schatzberg AF, Kraemer HC: Use of placebo control groups in evaluating efficacy of treatment of unipolar major depression. Biol Psychiatry 2000; 47:736-744

Thompson WG: Placebos: a review of the placebo response. Am J Gastroenterol 2000; 95:1637-1643

Chapter 11: References

Elenkov IJ, Iezzoni DG, Daly A, Harris AG, Chrousos GP (2005). "Cytokine dysregulation, inflammation and well-being". *Neuroimmunomodulation* 12 (5): 255 69.

Maruta T., Colligan R.C., Malinchoc M., and Offord K.P.: Optimists vs pessimists: survival rate among medical patients over a 30-year period. Mayo Clin Proc 2000; 75: pp. 140-143

Peterson C., Seligman M., and Valliant G.: Pessimistic explanatory style as a risk factor for physical illness: a thirty-five year longitudinal study. J Pers Soc Psychol 1988; 55: pp. 23-27.

Kamen-Siegel L., Rodin J., Seligman M.E., and Dwyer J.: Explanatory style and cell-mediated immunity in elderly men and women. Health Psychol 1991; 10: pp. 229-235.

Imai K., and Nakachi K.: Personality types, lifestyle, and sensitivity to mental stress in association with NK activity. Int J Hyg Environ Health 2001; 204: pp. 67-73.

Jung W., and Irwin M.: Reduction of natural killer cytotoxic activity in major depression: interaction between depression and cigarette smoking. Psychosom Med 1999; 61: pp. 263-270.

Kiecolt-Glaser J.K., McGuire L., Robles T.F., and Glaser R.: Emotions, morbidity, and mortality: new perspectives from psychoneuroimmunology. Annu Rev Psychol 2002; 53:

Kubera M, Maes M, Kenis G, Kim YK, Lasoń W (April 2005). "Effects of serotonin and serotonergic agonists and antagonists on the production of tumor necrosis factor alpha and interleukin-6". *Psychiatry Research* 134 (3): 251–8.

Kubera M, Lin AH, Kenis G, Bosmans E, van Bockstaele D, Maes M (April 2001). "Anti-Inflammatory effects of antidepressants through suppression of the interferon-gamma/interleukin-10 production ratio". *Journal of Clinical Psychopharmacology* 21 (2): 199–206.

Miller M, Fry W .(2009). Summary The effect of mirthful laughter on the human cardiovascular system. Med Hypotheses. Nov;73(5):636-9.

Provine R, Yong YL. Laughter: a stereotyped human vocalization. Ethology 1991;89:115–124.

Wild B, Rodden FA, Grodd W et al. Neural correlates of laughter and humour. Brain 2003;126:2121–2138.

Martin RA, Dobbin JP. Sense of humor, hassles, and immunoglobulin A: evidence for a stress-moderating effect of humor. Int J Psychiatry Med 1988;18:93–105.

Anderson C, Arnoult LH. An examination of perceived control, humor, irrational beliefs, and positive stress as moderators of the relation between negative stress and health. Basic Appl Soc Psych 1989;10:101–117.

Darwin C. The Expression of the Emotions in Man and Animals 3rd Ed. Oxford: Oxford University Press, 2002:1–512.

Lowdermilk D, Germino BB. Helping women and their families cope with the impact of gynecologic cancer. J Obstet Gynecol Neonatal Nurs 2000;29:653–660.

Joshua AM, Cotroneo A, Clarke S. Humor and oncology. J Clin Oncol 2005;23:645–648.
Fry W. Mirth and oxygen saturation levels of peripheral blood. Psychother and Psychosom. 1971;19:76–84.

Fry W. The physiological effects of humor, mirth, and laughter. J Am Med Assoc. 1992;267:1857–8.

Berk L, Tan S, Nehlsen-Cannarella S, Napier B, Lewis J, Lee J, et al. Humor associated laughter decreases cortisol and increases spontaneous lymphocyte blastogenesis. Clin Res. 1988;36:435A.

Berk L, Tan S, Napier B, Evy W. Eustress of mirthful laughter modifies natural killer cell activity. Clin Res. 1989;37:115A.

Berk L, Felten D, Tan S, Bittman, Westengard J. Modulation of neuroimmune parameters during the eustress of humor-associated mirthful laughter. Altern Ther Health Med. 2001;7:62–72. 74–6.

Seyle H. The general adaptation syndrome and the diseases of adaptation. J Clin Endocrinol Metab. 1946;6:117–230.

Nishida K, Hirota SK, Tokeshi J. (2008). Laugh syncope as a rare sub-type of the situational syncopes: a case report. J Med Case Reports Jun 7;2:197

Hayashi T, Tsujii S, Iburi T, Tamanaha T, Yamagami K, Ishibashi R, Hori M, Sakamoto S, Ishii H, Murakami K. 2007Laughter up-regulates the genes related to NK cell activity in diabetes. Biomed Res. 28(6):281-5.

Taylor S.E., Kemeny M.E., Reed G.M., et al: Psychological resources, positive illusions, and health. Am Psychol 2000; 55: pp. 99-109.

Schweizer K., Beck-Seyffer A., and Schneider R.: Cognitive bias of optimism and its influence on psychological well-being. Psychol Rep 1999; 84: pp. 627-636.

Chang E.C., and Sanna L.J.: Optimism, pessimism, and positive and negative affectivity in middle-aged adults: a test of a cognitive-affective model of psychological adjustment. Psychol Aging 2001; 16: pp. 524-531.

Segerstrom S.C.: Optimism, goal conflict, and stressor-related immune change. J Behav Med 2001; 24: pp. 441-467.

Chapter 12: References

Batkin S, Taussig SJ, and Szekerezes J (1988). Antimetastatic effect of bromelain with or without its proteolytic and anticoagulant activity. J Cancer Res Clin Oncol 114, 507 – 508.

Boivin GP, Washington K, Yang K, et al. (2003). Pathology of mouse models of intestinal cancer: consensus report and recommendations. Gastroenterology.;124:762–777.

Chichlowski M, Sharp JM, Vanderford DA, et al. (2008). Helicobacter typhlonius and H. rodentium differentially affect the severity of colon inflammation and inflammation-associated neoplasia in IL-10-deficient mice. Comp Med.;58:534–541.

Fitzhugh DJ, Shan S, Dewhirst MW, et al. (2008). Bromelain treatment decreases neutrophil migration to sites of inflammation. Clin Immunol.;128:66–74.

Fukushima Y, Ohnishi T, Arita N, Hayakawa T, and Sekiguchi K (1998). Integrin alpha3beta1 - mediated interaction with laminin – 5 stimulates adhesion, migration and invasion of malignant glioma cells. Int J Cancer 76, 63 – 72.

Giese A, and Westphal M (1996). Glioma invasion in the central nervous system. Neurosurgery 39, 235 – 250.

Hale LP, Greer PK, Trinh CT, et al. (2005). Treatment with oral bromelain decreases colonic inflammation in the IL-10-deficient murine model of inflammatory bowel disease. Clin Immunol.;116:135–142.

Kane S, Goldberg MJ. (2000). Use of bromelain for mild ulcerative colitis. Ann Int Med.;132:680.

Kleef R, Delohery TM, Bovbjerg DH. (1996). Selective modulation of cell adhesion molecules on lymphocytes by bromelain protease . Pathobiology.;64:339–346.

Onken JE, Greer PK, Calingaert B, et al. Bromelain treatment decreases secretion of pro-inflammatory cytokines and chemokines by colon biopsies in vitro. Clin Immunol. 2008;126:345–352.

Tysnes BB, Larsen LF, Ness GO, Mahesparan R, Edvardsen K, Garcia - Cabrera I, and Bjerkvig R (1996). Stimulation of glioma cell migration by laminin and inhibition by anti - alpha3 and anti - beta1 integrin antibodies. Int J Cancer 67, 777 – 784.

Tysnes BB, Haugland HK, and Bjerkvig R (1997). Epidermal growth factor and laminin receptors contribute to migratory and invasive properties of gliomas. Invasion Metastasis 17, 270 – 280.

Taussig SJ, Szekerczes J, and Batkin S (1985). Inhibition of tumour growth in vitro by bromelain, an extract of the pineapple plant (Ananas comosus). Planta Med 6, 538 – 539.

Uhm JH, Gladson CL, and Rao JS (1999). The role of integrins in the malignant phenotype of gliomas. Front Biosci 4, D188– D199.

Chapter 13: References

Wattenberg, L. Inhibition of carcinogenesis by minor dietary constituents. (1992). Cancer Res. (Suppl.), 52: 2085-2091.

Williams, D. E., Dashwood, R. H., Hendricks, J. D., and Bailey, G. S. (1990). Anticarcinogens and tumor promoters in foods. In: S. L. Taylor and R. A. Scanlan (eds.), Food Toxicology. A Perspective on the Relative Risks, pp.101-150.New York: Marcel Dekker, Inc.

Whitty, J. P., and Bjeldanes, L. F. (1987). The effects of dietary cabbage on xenobiotic metabolizing enzymes and binding of aflatoxin B, to hepatic DNA in rats. Food Chem. Toxicol., 25: 581-587.

McDanell, R., McLean, A. E. M., Hanley, A. B., Heaney, R. K., and Fenwick, G. R. (1988) Chemical and biological properties of indole glucosinolates (glucobrassicins): a review. Food Toxicol., 26: 59-70.

Bradfield, C. A., and Bjeldanes, L. F. (1987). Structure-activity relationships of dietary in doles: a proposed mechanism of action as modifiers of xenobiotic metabolism J. Toxicol. Environ. Health, 21: 311-323.

Vang, 0., Jensen, M. B., and Autrup, H. (1990). Induction of cytochrome P450 in rat colon and liver by indole-3-carbinol and 5,6-benzoflavone. Carcinogenesis (Lond.), *11: 1259-1263.*

Fong, A. T., Swanson, H. I., Dashwood, R. H., Williams, D. E., Hendricks, 1. D., andBailey, G. S. (1990). Mechanisms of anticarcinogenesis by indole-3-carbinol: studies of enzyme induction, electrophile-scavenging, and inhibition of aflatoxin B, activation. Biochem. Pharmacol., 39: 19-26.

Promotion of aflatoxin B, carcinogenesis by the natural tumor modulator indole-3-carbinol: influence of dose, duration, and intermittent exposure on indole-3-carbinol promotional potency. Cancer Res., 51: 2362-2365,1991.

Pence, B. C., Buddingh, F., and Yang, S. P. Multiple dietary factors in the enhancement of dimethylhydrazine carcinogenesis: main effect of indole-3-carbinol. J. Natl. Cancer Inst., 77: 269-276, 1986.

Rahman KM, Yiwei Li & Sarkar FH (2004). Inactivation of Akt and NF-κB Play Important Roles During Indole-3-Carbinol-Induced Apoptosis in Breast Cancer Cells. Nutrition and Cancer Vol.48,1, 84-94.

Chapter 14: References

Sikdar S, Mukherjee A, Khuda-Bukhsh AR. Anti-lung cancer potential of pure esteric-glycoside condurangogenin A against nonsmall-cell lung cancer cells in vitro via p21/p53 mediated cell cycle modulation and DNA damage-induced apoptosis. Pharmacogn Mag. 2015 May;11(Suppl 1):S73-85.

Khuda-Bukhsh AR, Sikdar S. Condurango 30C Induces Epigenetic Modification of Lung Cancer-specific Tumour Suppressor Genes via Demethylation. Forsch Komplementmed. 2015;22(3):172-9. doi: 10.1159/000433485.

Banerji P, Campbell DR, Banerji P. Cancer patients treated with the Banerji protocols utilising homoeopathic medicine: A Best Case Series Program of the National Cancer Institute USA. Oncol Rep. 2008;20:69–74.

Sikdar S, Mukherjee A, Boujedaini N, Khuda-Bukhsh AR. Ethanolic extract of condurango (*Marsdenia condurango*) used in traditional systems of medicine including homeopathy against cancer can induce DNA damage and apoptosis in nonsmall lung cancer cells, A549 and H522, *in vitro*. TANG Int J Genuine Tradit Med. 2013;3:1–10.

Sikdar S, Mukherjee A, Ghosh S, Khuda-Bukhsh AR. Condurango glycoside-rich components stimulate DNA damage-induced cell cycle arrest and ROS-mediated caspase-3 dependent apoptosis through inhibition of cell-proliferation in lung cancer, *in vitro* and *in vivo*. Environ Toxicol Pharmacol. 2014;37:300–14.

Fan W, Sun L, Zhou JQ, Zhang C, Qin S, Tang Y, et al. Marsdenia tenacissima extract induces G0/G1 cell cycle arrest in human esophageal carcinoma cells by inhibiting mitogen-activated protein kinase (MAPK) signaling pathway. Chin J Nat Med. (2015) 13:428–37.

To KKW, Wu X, Yin C, Chai S, Yao S, Kadioglu O, et al. Reversal of multidrug resistance by Marsdenia tenacissima and its main active ingredients polyoxypregnanes. J Ethnopharmacol. (2017) 203:110–9.

Jiang S, Qiu L, Li Y, Li L, Wang X, Liu Z, et al. Effects of Marsdenia tenacissima polysaccharide on the immune regulation and tumor growth in H22 tumor-bearing mice. Carbohydr Polym. (2016) 137:52–8.

Wang Y, Chen B, Wang Z, Zhang W, Hao K, Chen Y, et al. Marsdenia tenacissimae extraction (MTE) inhibits the proliferation and induces the apoptosis of human acute T cell leukemia cells through inactivating PI3K/AKT/mTOR signaling pathway via PTEN enhancement. Oncotarget (2016) 7:82851–63.

Dai X, Ji Y, Jiang P, Sun X. Marsdenia tenacissima extract suppresses tumor growth and angiogenesis in A20 mouse lymphoma. Oncol Lett. (2017) 13:2897–902.

Li D, Li C, Song Y, Zhou M, Sun X, Zhu X, et al. Marsdenia tenacssima extract and its functional components inhibits proliferation and induces apoptosis of human Burkitt leukemia/lymphoma cells in vitro and in vivo. Leuk Lymphoma. (2016) 57:419–28.

Ye B, Yang J, Li J, Niu T, Wang S. In vitro and in vivo antitumor activities of tenacissoside C from Marsdenia tenacissima. Planta Med. (2014b) 80:29–38.

Bode A, Dong Z. Apoptosis induction by arsenic: mechanisms of actions and possible clinical applications for treating therapy resistant cancers. J Drug Resist 2000; **3**:21–9.

Fisher DE. Apoptosis in cancer therapy: crossing the threshold. Cell 1994;78:539–42.

Rew DA. Cell and molecular mechanisms of pathogenesis and treatment of cancer. Postgrad Med J 1998;74:77–88

Staunton MJ, Gaffney EF. Apoptosis: basic concepts and potential significance in human cancer. Arch Pathol Lab Med 1998;122:310–9.

Steller H. Mechanisms and genes of cellular suicide. Science 1995;267:1445–9.

Sun HD, Ma L, Hu XC, Zhang TD. Ai-Lin I treated 32 cases of acute promyelocytic leukemia. Chin J Integrat Chinese Western Med 1992;12:170–2.

Chen GQ, Shi XG, Tang W, Xiong XM, Zhu J, Cai X, et al. Use of arsenic trioxide (As2O3) in the treatment of acute promyelocytic leukemia: I. As2O3 exerts dose-dependent dual effects on APL cells. Blood 1997;89:3345–53.

Gianni M, Koken MH, Chelbi-Alix MK, Benoit G, Lanotte M, Chen Z, et al. Combined arsenic and retinoic acid treatment enhances differentiation and apoptosis in arsenic-resistant NB4 cells. Blood 1998;91:4300.

Kitamura K, Yoshida H, Ohno R, Naoe T. Toxic effects of arsenic (As3+) and other metal ions on acute promyelocytic leukemia cells. Int J Hematol 1997;65:179–85.

Konig A, Wrazel L, Warrell RP Jr, Rivi R, Pandolfi PP, Jakubowski A, et al. Comparative activity of melarsoprol and arsenic trioxide in chronic B-cell leukemia lines. Blood 1997;90: 562–70.

Xin-Hua Zhu et al. Apoptosis and Growth Inhibition in Malignant Lymphocytes After Treatment With Arsenic Trioxide at Clinically Achievable Concentrations. Journal of the National Cancer Institute, Vol. 91, No. 9, May 5, 1999.

Zhang P, Wang SY, Hu XH. Arsenic trioxide treated 72 cases of acute promyelocytic leukemia. Chin J Hematol 1996;17:58–61.

Zhang W, Ohnishi K, Shigeno K, Fujisawa S, Naito K, Nakamura S, et al. The induction of apoptosis and cell cycle arrest by arsenic trioxide in lymphoid neoplasms. Leukemia 1998; 12:1383–91.

Falk MH, Meier T, Issels RD, Brielmeier M, Scheffer B, Bornkamm GW. Apoptosis in Burkitt lymphoma cells is prevented by promotion of cysteine uptake. Int J Cancer 1998;75: 620–5.

Lynn S, Shiung JN, Gurr JR, Jan KY. Arsenite stimulates poly(ADP-ribosylation) by generation of nitric oxide. Free Radic Biol Med 1998; 24:442–9.

Meng Z, Meng N. Effects of inorganic arsenicals on DNA synthesis in unsensitized human blood lymphocytes *in vitro*. Biol Trace Elem Res 1994;42:201–8.

Dai J, Weinberg RS, Waxman S, Jing Y. Malignant cells can be sensitized to undergo growth inhibition and apoptosis by arsenic trioxide through modulation of the glutathione redox system. Blood 1999;93:268–77.

Hale AL, Meepagala K, Oliva A, Aliotta G, Duke SO (2004). Phytotoxins from the Leaves of *Ruta graveolens*. J. Agric. Food Chem., 52: 3345-3349.

Ratheesh M, Helen A (2007). Anti-inflammatory activity of *Ruta graveolens* Linn on carrageenan induced paw edema in wistar male rats. Afr. J. Biotechnol., 6(10): 1209-1211.

Meepagala KM, Schrader KK, Wedge DE, Duke SO (2005). Algicidal and antifungal compounds from the roots of *Ruta graveolens* and synthesis of their analogs. Phytochemistry, 66: 2689-2695.

Pathak S, Multani AS, Banerji P, Banerji P (2003). Ruta 6 selectively induces cell death in brain cancer cells but proliferation in normal peripheral blood lymphocytes: A novel treatment for human brain cancer. Int. J. Oncol., 23: 975-982.

Schelz Z, Ocsovszki I, Bózsity N, Hohmann J, Zupkó I. Anti-proliferative Effects of Various Furanoacridones Isolated from Ruta graveolens on Human Breast Cancer Cell Lines. Anticancer Res. 2016 Jun;36(6):2751-8.

Ghosh S, Bishayee K, Khuda-Bukhsh AR. Graveoline isolated from ethanolic extract of Ruta graveolens triggers apoptosis and autophagy in skin melanoma cells: a novel apoptosis-independent autophagic signaling pathway. Phytother Res. 2014 Aug;28(8):1153-62.

Fadlalla K, Watson A, Yehualaeshet T, Turner T, Samuel T. Ruta graveolens extract induces DNA damage pathways and blocks Akt activation to inhibit cancercell proliferation and survival. Anticancer Res. 2011 Jan;31(1):233-41.

Varamini P, Soltani M, Ghaderi A. Cell cycle analysis and cytotoxic potential of Ruta graveolens against human tumor cell lines. Neoplasma. 2009;56(6):490-3.

Chapter 15: References

Hayakawa H, Minaniya Y, Ito K, Yamamoto, Fukuda T. Difference of curcumin content in Curcuma longa L. (Zingiberaceae) caused by hybridization with other Curcuma species. *Am J Plant Sci.* 2011;2(2):111–119.

Annadurai RS, Neethiraj R, Jayakumar V, et al. De Novo Transcriptome Assembly (NGS) of Curcuma longa L. Rhizome Reveals Novel Transcripts Related to Anticancer and Antimalarial Terpenoids. *PLoS One.* 2013;8:56217.

Ammon H, Wahl MA. Pharmacology of Curcuma longa. *Planta Med.* 1991;57(1):1–7.

Schraufstätter E, Bernt H. Antibacterial action of curcumin and related compounds. *Nature.* 1949;164(4167):456.

Srimal RC, Dhawan BN. Pharmacology of diferuloyl methane (curcumin), a non-steroidal anti-inflammatory agent. *J Pharm Pharmacol.* 1973;25(6): 447–452.

Sharma OP. Antioxidant activity of curcumin and related compounds. *Biochem Pharmacol.* 1976;25(15):1811–1812.

Shehzad A, Lee YS. Molecular mechanisms of curcumin action: Signal transduction. *Biofactors.* 2013;39(1):27–36.

Singh S, Khar A. Biological effects of curcumin and its role in cancer chemoprevention and therapy. *Anticancer Agents Med Chem.* 2006;6(3):259–70.

Kuttan R, Bhanumathy P, Nirmala K, George MC. Potential anticancer activity of turmeric

(Curcuma longa). *Cancer Lett.* 1985;29(2):197–202.

Kuttan R, Sudheeran PC, Josph CD. Turmeric and curcumin as topical agents in cancer therapy. *Tumori.* 1987;73(1):29–31.

Bayet-Robert M, Kwiatkowski F, Leheurteur M, et al. Phase I dose escalation trial of docetaxel plus curcumin in patients with advanced and metastatic breast cancer. *Cancer Biol Ther.* 2010;9(1):8–14.

Carroll RE, Benya RV, Turgeon DK, et al. Phase IIa clinical trial of curcumin for the prevention of colorectal neoplasia. *Cancer Prev Res (Phila).* 2011;4(3):354–364.

Bussolino, F., Mantovani, A., and Persico, G. Molecular mechanisms of blood vessel formation. Trends Biochem. Sci., *22:* 251–256, 1997.

Singh J, Dubey RK, Ata CK I (1986). "Piperine-mediated inhibition of glucuronidation activity in isolated epithelial cells of the guinea-pig small intestine: evidence that piperine lowers the endogeneous UDP-glucuronic acid content". Pharamcol. Exp. Ther.236: 488–493.

Suzuki, T., and Iwai, K. Constitution of red pepper species: chemistry, biochemistry, pharmacology, and food science of the pungent principle of Capsicum species. *In:* A. Brosi, Ed., The Alkaloides, pp. 227–299. New York: Academic Press, 1994.

Cordell, G. A., and Araujo, O. E. Capsaicin: identification, nomenclature, and pharmacotherapy. Ann. Pharmacother., *27:* 330–336, 1993.

Surh, Y. J., Lee, E., and Lee, J. M. Chemopreventive properties of some pungent ingredients present in red pepper and ginger. Mutat. Res., *402:* 259–267, 1998.

Morre, D. J., Chuen, P. J., and Morre, D. M. Capsaicin inhibits preferentially the NADH oxidase and growth of transformed cells in culture. Proc. Natl. Acad. Sci. USA, *92:* 1831–1835, 1995.

Kim, J. D., Kim, J. M., Pyo, J. O., Kim, S. Y., Kim, B. S., Yu, R., and Han, I. S. Capsaicin can alter the expression of tumor forming-related genes which might be followed by induction of apoptosis of a Korean stomach cancer cell line, SNU-1. Cancer Lett., *120:* 235–241, 1997.

Szallasi, A., and Blumberg, P. M. Vanilloid (Capsaicin) receptors and mechanisms. Pharmacol. Rev., *51:* 159–212, 1999.

Archer, V. E., and Jones, D. W. Capsaicin pepper, cancer and ethnicity. Med. Hyp., *59:* 450–457, 2002.

McMahon, G. VEGF Receptor signaling in tumor angiogenesis. Oncologist, *5:* 3–10, 2000.

www.ingramcontent.com/pod-product-compliance
Lightning Source LLC
Chambersburg PA
CBHW071354210526
45465CB00001B/85